跟医生认常用穴位

（双语手绘版）

Learn Common Acupoints from Doctors

（ *Bilingual and Hand-painted Version* ）

主 编　陈 华　齐昌菊　郁东海

Editor　Chen Hua　Qi Changju　Yu Donghai

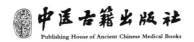

中医古籍出版社
Publishing House of Ancient Chinese Medical Books

图书在版编目（CIP）数据

跟医生认常用穴位：双语手绘版：汉、英 / 陈华，齐昌菊，郁东海主编 . — 北京：中医古籍出版社，2024.1

ISBN 978-7-5152-2564-7

Ⅰ . ①跟⋯　Ⅱ . ①陈⋯　②齐⋯　③郁⋯　Ⅲ . ①穴位—介绍—汉、英　Ⅳ . ① R224.2

中国版本图书馆 CIP 数据核字（2022）第 166386 号

跟医生认常用穴位：双语手绘版

主编　陈　华　齐昌菊　郁东海

策划编辑　郑　蓉

责任编辑　李美玲

文字编辑　王安琪

责任校对　吕　明

封面设计　李　绮

出版发行　中医古籍出版社

社　　址　北京市东城区东直门内南小街 16 号（100700）

电　　话　010-64089446（总编室）010-64002949（发行部）

网　　址　www.zhongyiguji.com.cn

印　　刷　北京市泰锐印刷有限责任公司

开　　本　880mm×1230mm　1/16

印　　张　5.5

字　　数　105 千字

版　　次　2024 年 1 月第 1 版　2024 年 1 月第 1 次印刷

书　　号　ISBN 978-7-5152-2564-7

定　　价　58.00 元

《跟医生认常用穴位》编委会

主编
陈华 [1,2]　齐昌菊 [1]　郁东海 [3]

执行主编
李萍 [1]　王瑾 [1]　侯坤 [1]

副主编
黄奏琴 [2]　赵志国 [4]　杨冠男 [5]

执行副主编
李华章 [1]　赵春燕 [1]　齐佳龙 [2]

主审
吴耀持 [6]

编委
都乐亦 [7]　邓镇荡 [8]　冯欣茵 [9]　仇万兴 [2]　苏齐 [9]
吴勤 [7]　杨睿 [1]　周辉霞 [10]　张玲玲 [1]

翻译
兰蕾 [11]

漫画·设计
李琦 [12]

参编人员单位
1.上海市浦东新区光明中医医院
2.上海市浦东新区中医医院
3.上海市浦东新区卫生健康委员会
4.上海中医药大学附属上海市中西医结合医院
5.首都医科大学附属北京康复医院
6.上海交通大学附属第六人民医院
7.上海市浦东新区中医药创新促进中心
8.湖南省浏阳市集里医院
9.上海养和堂中医门诊部
10.广州荔湾固元堂中医门诊部
11.上海市浦东卫生发展研究院
12.上海昂悦建筑装饰工程有限公司

编 者 序

2017年7月1日，《中华人民共和国中医药法》正式实施。其中指出，"加强中医药文化宣传，普及中医药知识，鼓励组织和个人创作中医药文化和科普作品"，支持和鼓励中医药科普。

现在市面上有很多针灸穴位方面的书籍，大部分都使用了大量的文字、非常专业的语言，很难被中老年读者理解，如何打破这些普及传播中医药知识遇到的障碍，是摆在中医科普传播从业者面前的一道难题。

基于以上思考，作者选择用简单明了的手绘漫画来传递古老中医药文化知识的精髓，让生涩深奥的理论知识变为浅显易懂、跃然纸上的漫画。而且，读者可以通过高清拍摄的穴位图片快速找到准确位置，并且跟随漫画医生示范的方法，推拿或者灸法刺激穴位，达到缓解身体不适、防病治病的目的。

本书按头面颈部、胸腹部、四肢部分为3章，共计38个穴位。书中采用高清拍摄图片加手绘的形式，让朋友们更好地理解穴位的魅力，充满了趣味性和科学性，让中老年读者在理解穴位知识的同时，还可以学习简单的方法为自己防病治病。英语部分增加了书本的实用性，让这本书能够跨越时空的界限，跨越语言的障碍，将中医药文化传播到世界各地。

本书由上海市浦东新区光明中医医院牵头编写，获得了2019年度浦东新区"国家中医药发展综合改革试验区"建设项目(编号：PDZY-2019-0811)立项资助，得到了上海中医药大学、浦东新区卫生与健康委员会中医药发展与科教处、浦东新区中医药发展中心、浦东新区中医药创新促进中心等单位的大力协助。本书虽然经过多次修订，但内容可能还有不少疏漏，真诚希望各位读者能够斧正。

编者

2021年12月

目录 **Contents**

头面颈部穴位

胸腹部穴位

四肢部穴位

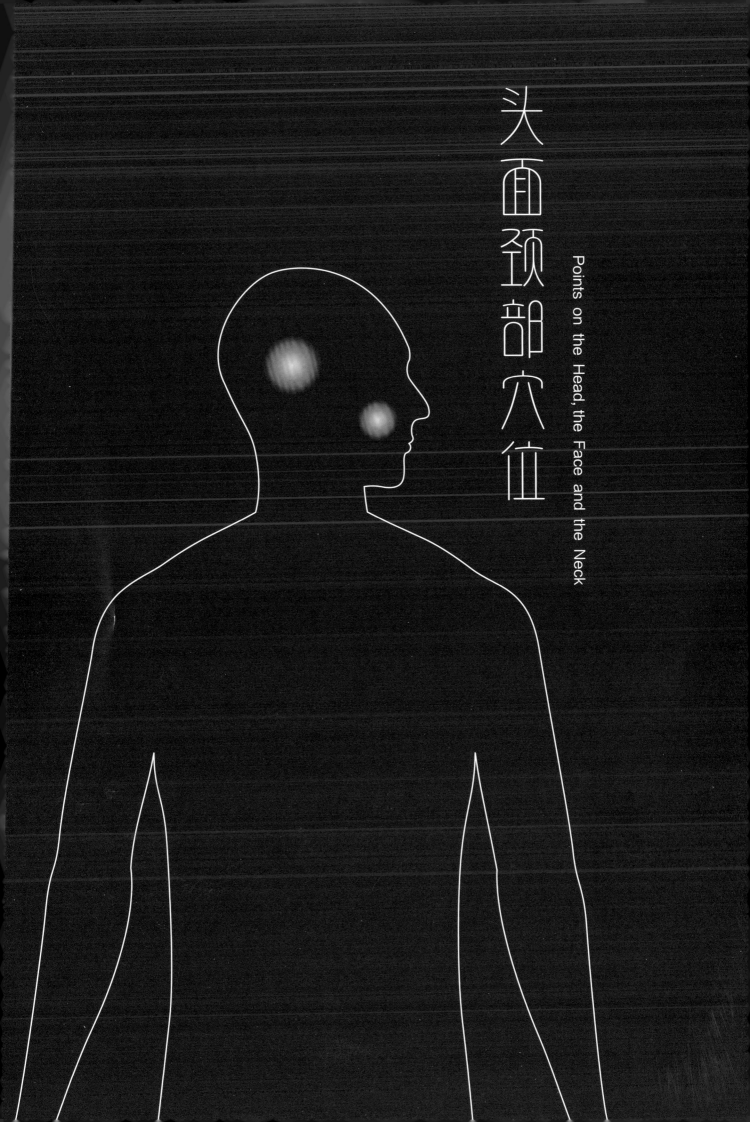

头面颈部穴位

Points on the Head, the Face and the Neck

百会穴

| 来　源 | 本穴处于人之头顶，在人体的最高处，人体各经上传的阳气都交会于此，故名百会。 |

| 位　置 | 位于头顶正中线与两耳尖连线的交点处。 |

| 主要作用 | 治疗头痛、头重脚轻、目眩、高血压、低血压、宿醉、痔疮、失眠、焦躁等。此穴为人体督脉上的重要穴位之一，是治疗多种疾病的首选穴，医学研究价值很高。 |

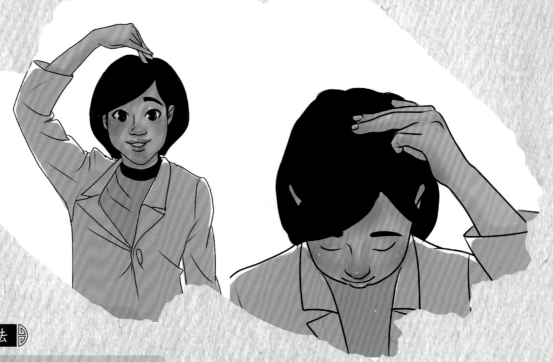

| 操作方法 |

以一手的中指或食指附于百会穴上，先由轻渐重地按3～5下，然后再顺时针、逆时针各旋转揉动30～50次。如果是体质虚弱或患有内脏下垂、脱肛等症的朋友，开始按揉时动作要轻一些，以后逐渐加重，按摩的次数也可随之增多。

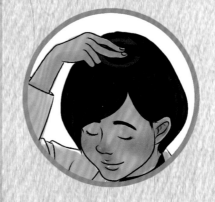 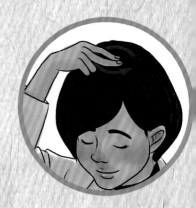

Baihui Point (DU20)

Nomenclature   Baihui is located at the top of the head where yang qi of all meridians goes upwards and meets here.

Location   At the midpoint of the line connecting the apexes of the two auricles.

Indications   Headache, heavy sensation of the head, vertigo, hypertension,hypotension, hangover, haemorrhoids, insomnia, anxiety and restlessness. As an important point in Du Meridian, it is the first choice for treating many diseases.

Methods   Press the point gently and then forcefully for 3 to 5 times with middle finger or index finger. Next, rub in a circular motion clockwise and anticlockwise each for 30 to 50 times. If you are weak or diagnosed with visceral ptosis or rectocele, rub it gently first. Add the force and frequency gradually.

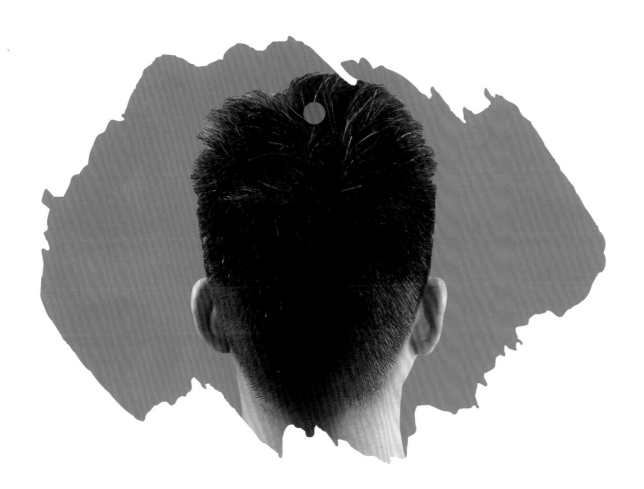

印堂穴

来源 古人将额部两眉头之间称为"阙"，星象家称之为印堂，故取此名。

位置 位于人体的面部，两眉头连线中点。

主要作用 治疗头痛、前头痛、失眠、高血压、鼻塞、流涕、头晕眼花等。

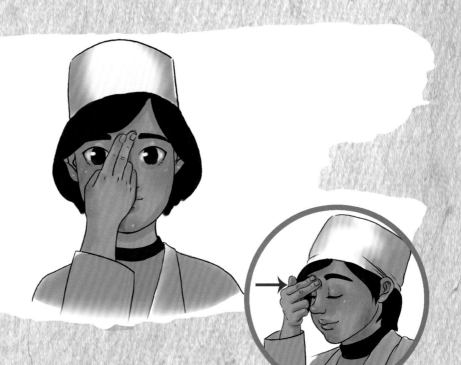

操作方法

按摩时可以用大拇指指腹轻揉，回旋按摩，力度要适中，不可深力度按压，每天施治时间3～5分钟，每日2～3次。或用拇指或食指、中指的指腹按压印堂穴12次，也可以用两手中指一左一右交替按摩印堂穴。此法可以刺激嗅觉细胞，使嗅觉灵敏，还能预防感冒和呼吸道疾病。

Yintang Point (DU29)

Nomenclature   The area between the eyebrows is called Que (阙), which is also known as Yintang by astrologers.

Location   On the forehead, at the midpoint between the two medial ends of the eyebrows.

Indications   Headache, frontal pain, insomnia, hypertension, nasal congestion, running nose, dizziness, blurred vision.

Methods   Rub the point in a circular motion moderately with the pulp of the thumb for 2 to 3 times a day with 3 to 5 minutes each time. Or, press the point with the pulp of thumb, index finger or middle finger for 12 times. Or, rub it with middle fingers, respectively. This method can enhance the proliferation of epithelial cells of nasal mucous membrane, stimulate olfactory cell and make the sense of smell sharp. In addition, it can prevent cold and respiratory diseases.

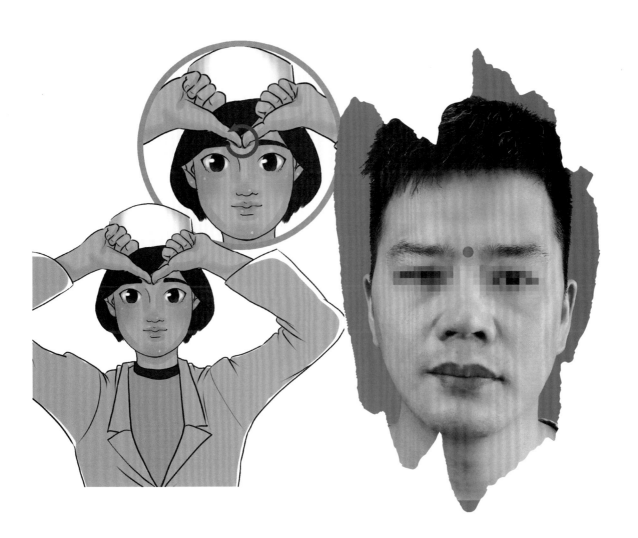

睛明穴

来源 名意指眼睛接受膀胱经的气血而变得明亮。

位置 位于面部，目内眦角稍上方凹陷处。

主要作用 　　睛明穴是治疗眼部疾病常用的穴位之一，尤其对于经常用眼的人士来讲，更应该熟练准确地掌握此穴的取穴方法，只要简单地按摩一会儿，就可以明显地缓解眼部疲劳。对于学生而言，此穴更是不可多得的预防近视的穴位之一。

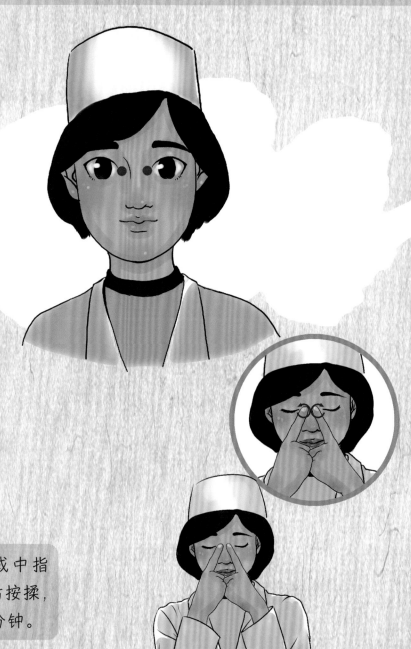

操作方法

　　用食指或中指指腹轻点住后按揉，每穴2～3分钟。

Jingming Point (BL1)

Nomenclature The point indicates that the eyes become bright after receiving the qi and blood of Bladder Meridian.

Location On the face, in the depression superior to the inner canthus.

Indications Jingming point is commonly used. Those who use eyes frequently are advised to master how to locate the point. Rubbing for 1 to 2 minutes can significantly relax your eyes.The point can also be used for preventing nearsightedness, especially for students.

Methods Press and rub the point with the pulp of index finger or middle finger for 2 to 3 minutes.

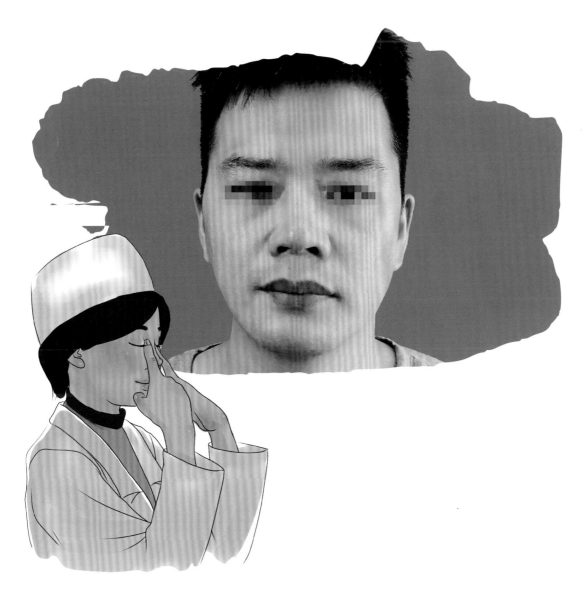

7

太阳穴

来源 经外奇穴，古人将眉梢后、鬓角前的穴位称为太阳穴。

位置 目外眦与眉梢连线中点向后外一横指，可触及一凹陷，用力按压有明显酸胀感即是本穴。

主要作用 治疗头痛、偏头痛、眼睛疲劳、牙痛等。当人们长时间连续用脑后，太阳穴往往会出现重压或胀痛的感觉，这就是大脑疲劳的信号。这时施以按摩效果会非常显著。按摩太阳穴可以给大脑以良性刺激，能够解除疲劳、振奋精神、止痛醒脑，并且能帮助人们继续保持注意力的集中。

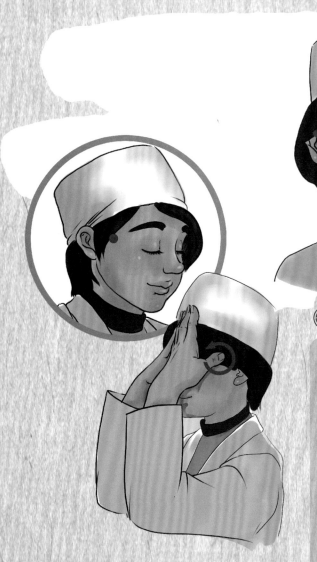

操作方法

将手掌搓热，贴于太阳穴，稍稍用力，顺时针转揉10～20次，再逆时针转揉相同的次数。也可以将手掌贴在额头上，以拇指指腹分别按在两边的太阳穴上，稍用力使太阳穴微感疼痛，然后，顺时针、逆时针各转揉相同的次数。一般按摩的次数可多可少，可以自己按照大脑疲劳的程度调整。

Taiyang Point (EX-HN5)

Nomenclature　It is an extraordinary point. Ancient people call the point located between the outer end of the eyebrow and the temple as Taiyang point.

Location　In the region of the temples, in the depression about one finger-breadth posterior to the midpoint between the lateral end of the eyebrow and the outer canthus.

Indications　Headache, migraine, eye strain, toothache and so on. When people think continuously for a long time, Taiyang point will have a heavy sensation or swelling pain, indicating fatigue in the brain. At this time, apply tuina on this point will be effective in relieving the fatigue and pain, making you refreshing and improve your focus.

Methods　Rub the palm until it becomes suffused with warmth. Next, put the palm on the Taiyang point with moderate force and then knead clockwise for 10 to 20 times and then anticlockwise for 10 to 20 times. Or, put the palms on the head and press the points with moderate force with the pulp of the thumb.The frequency should be adjusted based on the degree of the brain fatigue.

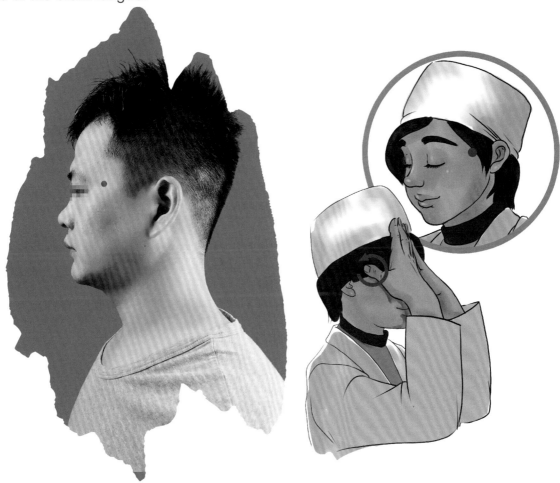

迎香穴

来　源	此穴在鼻旁，因能治疗鼻塞闻不出气味，故名。
位　置	用手指沿鼻唇沟向上推，至鼻翼中点旁，可触及一凹陷，即是本穴。
主要作用	治疗鼻塞、鼻子出血、面瘫口歪等。

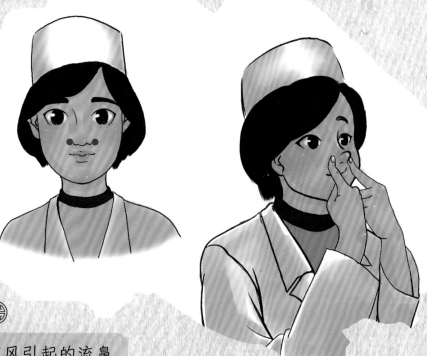

操作方法

如有伤风引起的流鼻涕、鼻塞，或者过敏性鼻炎，患者局部涂抹润滑油后，按摩迎香至发热，能缓解症状。经常用食指指腹垂直按压迎香，每次1～3分钟，能使鼻子保持舒畅，对肺部也有很好的保健作用，可预防肺系疾病。

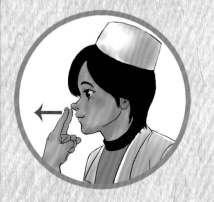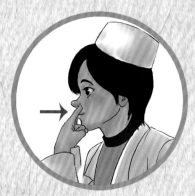

Yingxiang Point (LI20)

Nomenclature　Located at the border of the ala nasi, the point can treat the patient who cannot smell the fragrance with nasal congestion. That's why the point is named Yingxiang (English translation: welcome fragrance).

Location　At the midpoint lateral to the border of the ala nasi, in the nasolabial groove.

Indications　Nasal congestion, epistaxis, facioplegia etc.

Methods　The patient with running nose, nasal congestion induced by common colds or allergic rhinitis can rub Yingxiang points to relieve the symptoms. After putting some lubricants on the points, you can rub them with your index fingers until you feel warm. Meanwhile, you can also press the points perpendicularly for 1 to 3 minutes each time to keep the nose function well and prevent lung diseases.

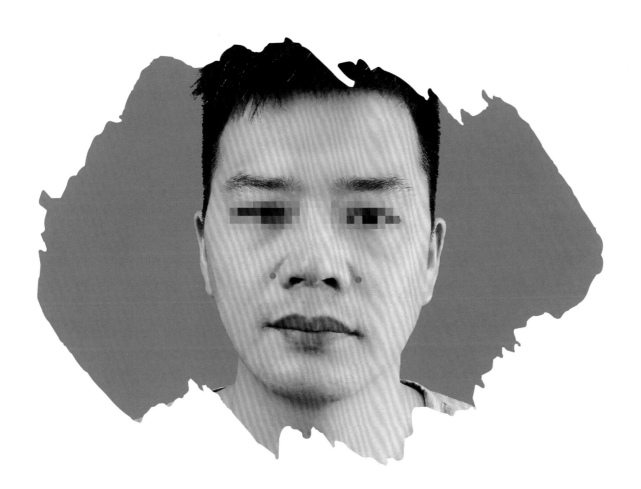

四白穴

来　源　意指胃经经水在本穴快速气化成为天部之气，气化之气形成白雾之状充斥四周，且清晰可见。

位　置　在面部，双眼平视时，瞳孔直下，当眶下孔凹陷处。

主要作用　本穴明目效果非常显著。对于上学的孩子，它可以用来治疗近视；对于中年人，它可以用来防止黑眼圈；对于老年人，它还可以用来防止老花眼。

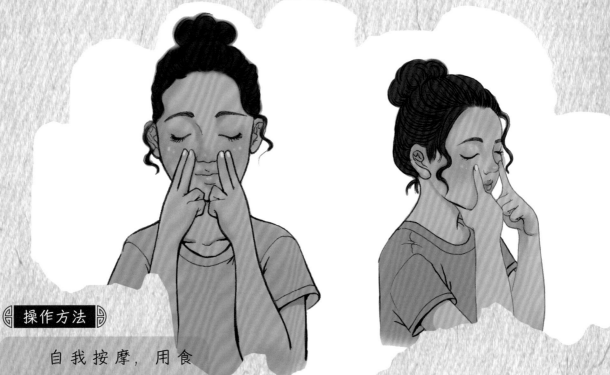

操作方法

　　自我按摩，用食指指腹轻轻揉按此穴，旋转按揉1圈为1拍，如做8个8拍即64拍，则每过1个8拍就改变1次旋转方向。动作要领：手指相对穴位表面不需要移动，按揉面不要太大。

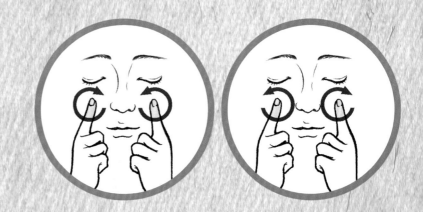

Sibai Point (ST2)

Nomenclature Meridian water of Stomach Meridian quickly vaporizes into heaven qi which looks like fog and can be seen everywhere.

Location On the face, the point is directly below the pupil of the eye, in the depression at the infraorbital foramen.

Indications Sibai point is effective in promoting the vision. Kneading the point can guide qi and blood into the eye. It can be used to treat nearsightedness, dark circles and farsightedness.

Methods Gently rub the point with your index finger for 64 circles. Rub in 8 circles clockwise and then 8 circles anticlockwise. Keep your index finger fixed on the point while rubbing gently.

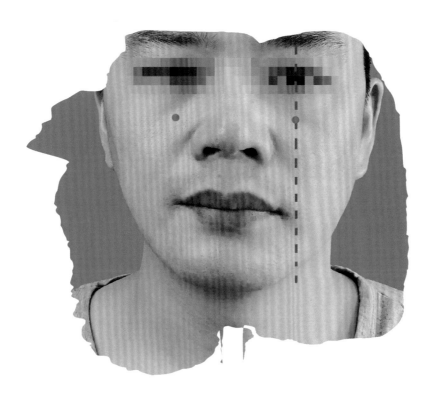

13

水沟穴

来　源	穴在鼻柱下，因喻穴处犹如涕水之沟渠，故名。
位　置	位于人中沟正中线上三分之一与三分之二交界处，用力按压有酸胀感。
主要作用	主治昏迷、晕厥、惊厥抽搐、口干等多种病症，为中医抢救危重病人的急救穴之一。

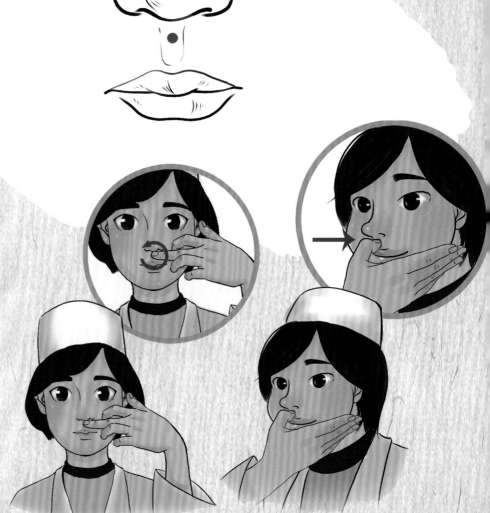

操作方法

用食指或中指指腹按揉此穴，或以拇指甲角代针掐压水沟穴，施以强刺激手法，昏迷病人将会苏醒。注意本穴不灸。

Shuigou Point (DU26)

Nomenclature   The point is below the nose and in the philtrum, which looks like a water groove.

Location   On the face, at the junction of the superior 1/3 and middle 1/3 of the philtrum. Press the point and you'll fell sore and swollen.

Indications   Coma, syncope, eclampsia, convulsion, dry mouth and so on. The point is often used to rescue the critically ill patients in an emergency.

Methods   Press and rub the point with the pulp of index finger or middle finger. Or, pinch the point with the sharp part of the thumbnail. The strong stimulation will waken the patients. Moxibustion cannot be applied to this point.

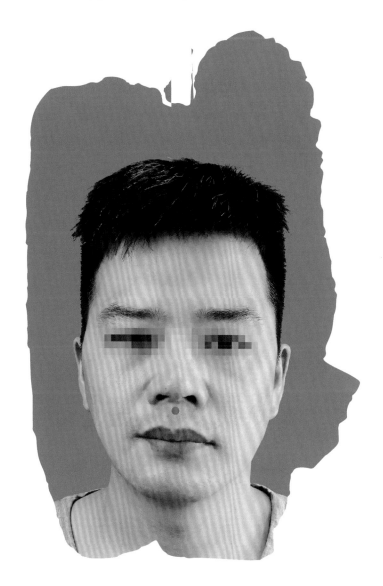

15

地仓穴

来　源	地，脾胃之土也；仓，五谷存储聚散之所也，国家之粮库。
位　置	位于人体面部，口角外侧，上直对瞳孔。
主要作用	地仓穴对于流涎、口角发炎、三叉神经痛有很好的疗效。

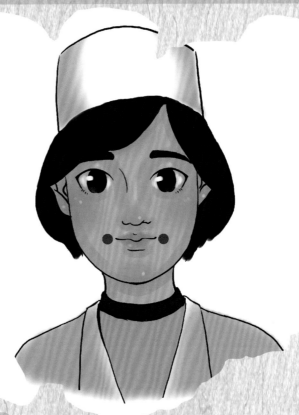

操作方法

用艾条灸3~5分钟，局部有热感即可，避免烫伤。按摩也是可以的，按摩本穴力度适中为好，尤其给孩子按摩的时候要注意不可以太用力。每次施治时间为3~5分钟，每天3次左右。

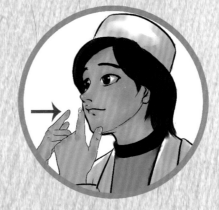 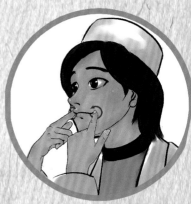

Dicang Point (ST4)

Nomenclature   Di indicates the spleen and stomach which pertains to the earth; Cang means the granary where grains are stored.

Location   On the face, lateral to the corner of the mouth, directly below the pupil of the eye.

Indications   Dicang is the best point to treat salivation, angular cheilitis and trigeminal neuralgia.

Methods   Hold a burning moxa stick close to the point for 3 to 5 minutes until the patient feels warm. Be careful and avoid burns. Tuina is also feasible. You can gently rub the point, especially for children, 3 times a day for 3 to 5 minutes each time.

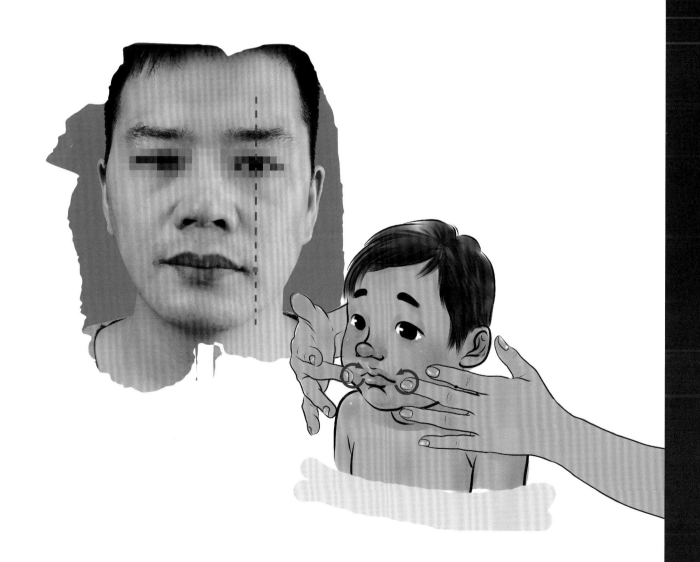

下关穴

来　源　　意指本穴对上输头部的气血中的阴浊部分及气血精微有关卡、把关的作用。

位　置　　由耳屏前向前一横指可触及一高骨，即为颧弓，颧弓下方的凹陷处就是本穴，张口时会隆起。

主要作用　　常用于治疗下颌关节炎、三叉神经痛、牙痛、嘴歪、斜视等病症，以及耳聋、耳鸣、耳道流脓等耳疾。

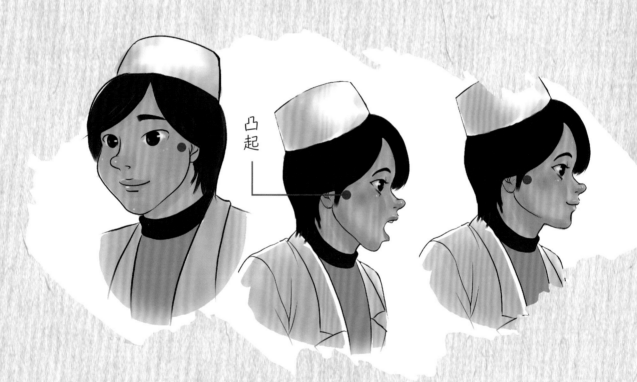

凸起

操作方法

用拇指向牙根部按压为主，中等力度使局部酸胀。

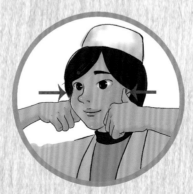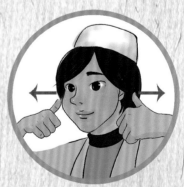

Xiaguan Point (ST7)

Nomenclature The point guards the pass where turbidity and essence in qi and blood flow up into the head.

Location On the face, anterior to the ear, in the depression below the zygomatic arch. The point is bulged when the mouth is opened and depressed when the mouth is closed.

Indications The point is used to treat mandibular arthritis, trigeminal neuralgia, toothache,deviated mouth and eyes, deafness, tinnitus, ear infection and so on.

Methods Press the point towards gingiva with your thumb moderately until the area feels sore and swelling.

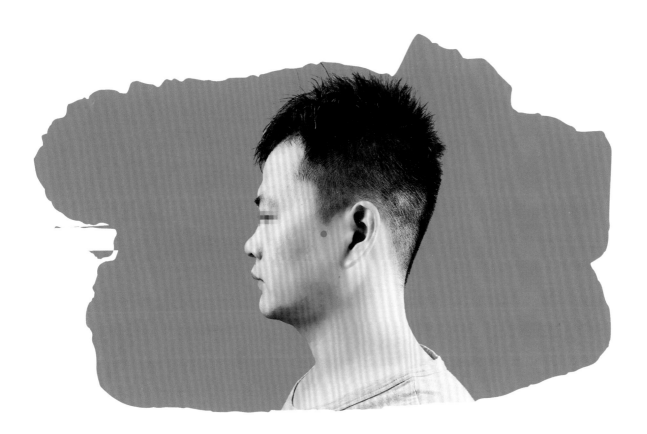

风池穴

来源 由脑空穴传来的水湿之气，至本穴后，因受外部之热，水湿之气胀散并化为阳热风气输散于头颈各部，故名风池。

位置 后头骨下两条大筋的外缘有两凹陷，大致与耳垂齐平，用力按压有酸胀感，即是本穴。

主要作用 治疗头痛、头重脚轻、眼睛疲劳、颈部酸痛、落枕、失眠等。

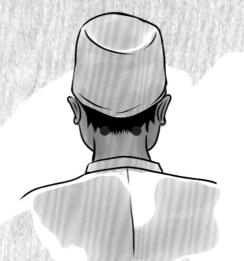

操作方法

以两手食指、中指指腹，紧按风池穴，用力旋转按揉几下，随后按揉脑后，做30次左右，以有酸胀感为宜，此法具有安神催眠的疗效。

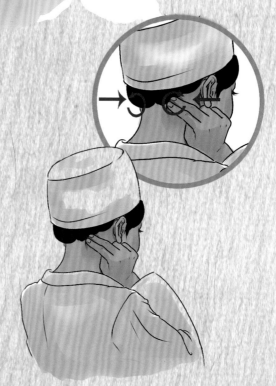

Fengchi Point (GB20)

Nomenclature The water and dampness arrive at the point and then get heated by the external heat. After vaporizing, the qi of water and dampness transforms into warm wind that is distributed on the head and neck.

Location At the meeting-place of the base of the skull and top of the neck, just lateral to the tendons of the trapezius muscle, at the level of the earlobe. Press the point and you'll feel sore and swollen.

Indications Fengchi is the main point for diseases like headache, heavy sensation of the head, eye strain, soreness and pain of the neck, stiff neck and insomnia.

Methods Press the point with your index and middle fingers, then rub it in a circular motion with force.Then rub the back of the head for 30 times until you feel sore and swollen. This method is effective in tranquillizing and promoting sleep.

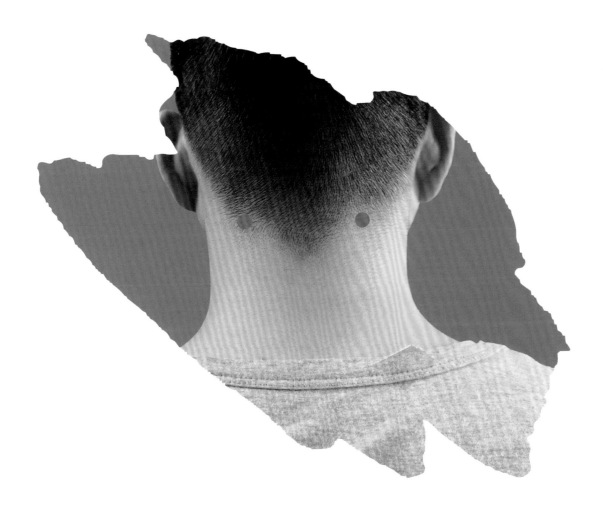

21

大椎穴

来源 穴内的阳气充足满盛如椎般坚实，故名大椎。

位置 位于第7颈椎棘突下凹陷中。（特别说明：后正中线上可见颈部和背部交界处有一高突的骨头，这个骨头可以随颈部左右摆动而转动，它就是第7颈椎。）

主要作用 治疗感冒、后脑勺和脖子痛、小儿抽搐、小儿麻痹后遗症等。

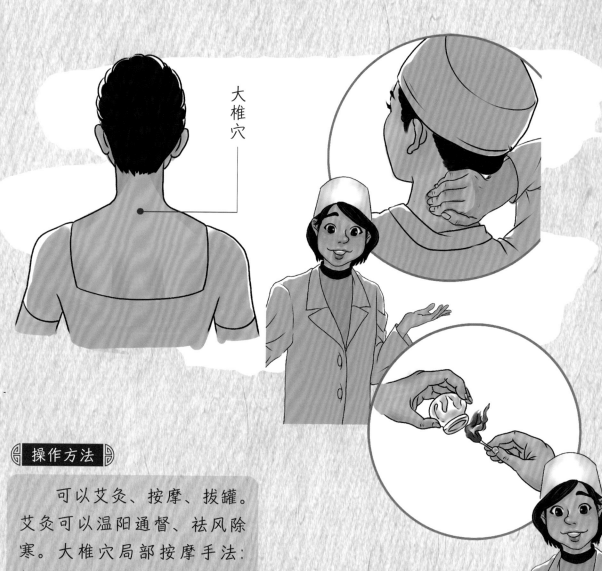

大椎穴

操作方法

可以艾灸、按摩、拔罐。艾灸可以温阳通督、祛风除寒。大椎穴局部按摩手法：如颈项部酸胀不适，可以用揉法、擦法、拍法等。

Dazhui Point (DU14)

Nomenclature   Dazhui is filled with yang qi which makes this point as strong as a vertebra.

Location   On the posterior median line, in the depression below the spinous process of the 7th cervical vertebra. At the border between the back and neck, this spinous process can be easily found, as it rotates when you turn your face to the sides.

Indications   Common cold, pain in the back of the head, neck pain; convulsion and polio aftereffects.

Methods   Moxibustion, tuina and cupping therapy can be applied. Moxibustion can free Du Meridian by warming yang, dispel wind and cold. Tuina can also be used for stiff or sore neck, such as rubbing, kneading and patting.

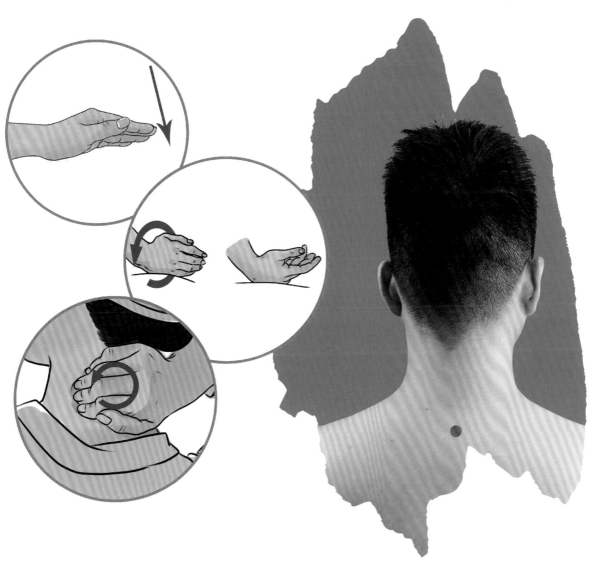

胸腹部穴位

Points on the Chest and the Abdomen

天突穴

来　源	意指任脉气血在此吸热后突行上天。
位　置	位于颈部，当前正中线上，胸骨上窝中央。
主要作用	治疗支气管哮喘、支气管炎、甲状腺肿大、食道炎、失声、口吐脓血、咽喉肿痛、慢性咽炎等。

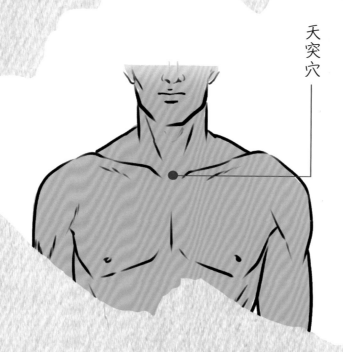

天突穴

操作方法

自我点按或按揉，可用中指指腹按揉或点按，一般顺时针按揉50～100次。

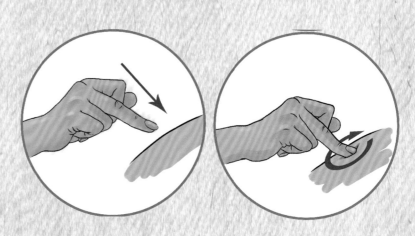

Tiantu Point (RN22)

Nomenclature   Qi and blood of Ren Meridian absorb heat here and then sharply flow up to the heaven.

Location   On the anterior median line of the neck, in the center of the suprasternal fossa.

Indications   Bronchial asthma, bronchitis, thyromegaly, esophagitis, aphonia, vomiting pus and blood, sore throat, chronic pharyngitis.

Methods   Press and rub Tiantu point clockwise for 50 to 100 circles with the pulp of middle finger.

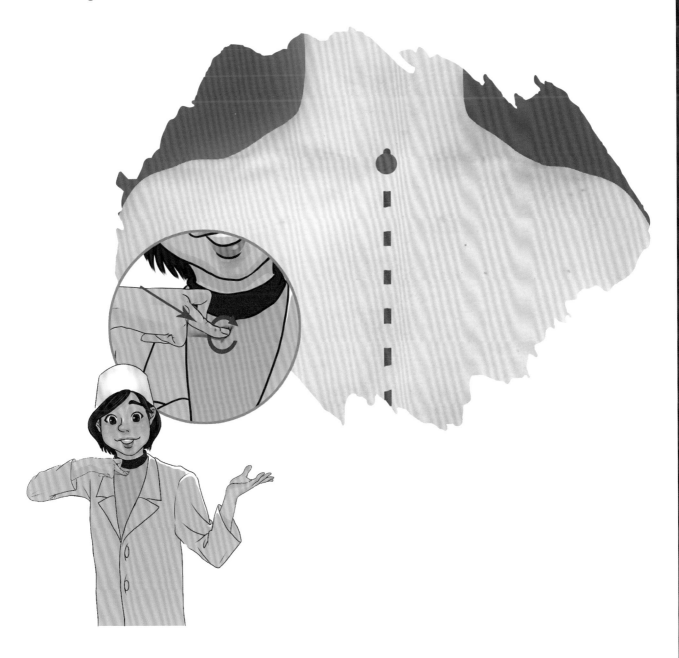

膻中穴

来　源	《灵枢·胀论》云"膻中者，心主之宫城也"，盖指心包膜部位而言。本穴内景，正应心包外腔，故名膻中。
位　置	在前正中线上，两乳头连线的中点。
主要作用	治疗胸部胀满不适或疼痛，腹部疼痛，心慌胸闷等。

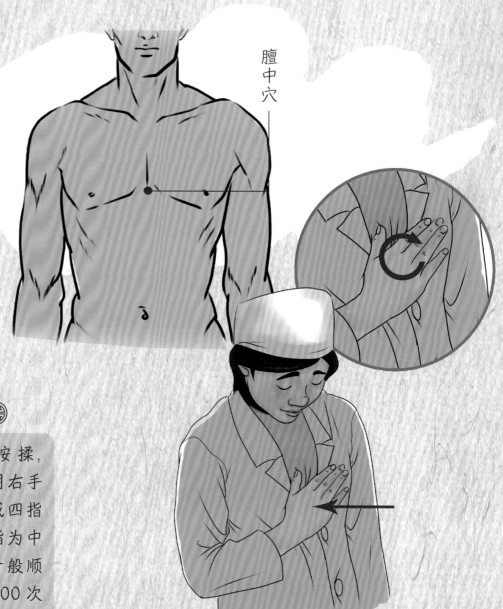

膻中穴

操作方法

自我按揉，按揉时可用右手大鱼际，或四指并拢以中指为中心按揉，一般顺时针按揉100次左右。

Danzhong Point (RN17)

Nomenclature According to *Lingshu Zhanglun* (*Spiritual Pivot. On Distension*), Danzhong is the palace where the heart lives in, about referring to the pericardium. The point exactly corresponds to the external pericardium.

Location On the anterior median line of the chest, at the midpoint between the two nipples.

Indications Pain and oppression of the chest, abdominal pain, palpitations.

Methods Press and rub Danzhong point clockwise for 100 circles with the thenar eminence or the middle finger (with four fingers close to each other).

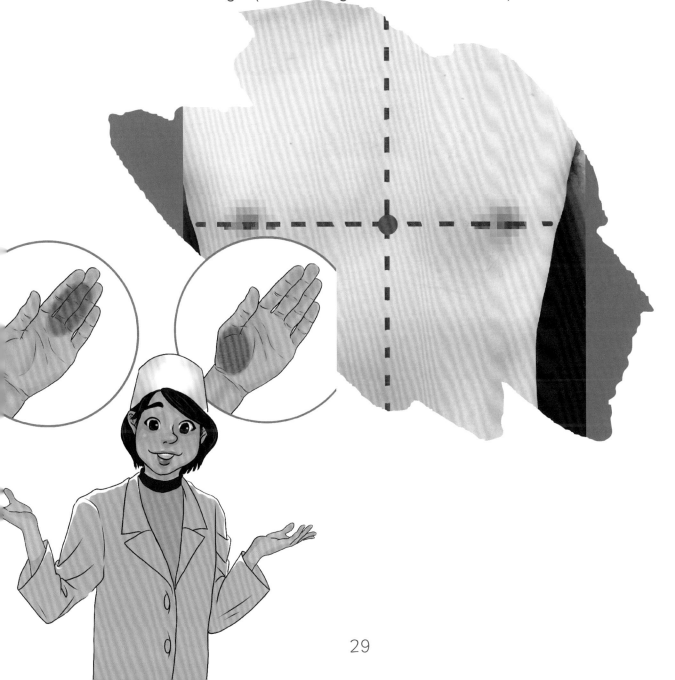

中脘穴

来　源　中，指本穴相对于上脘穴、下脘穴二穴而为中也。

位　置　位于人体上腹部，前正中线上，当脐中上4寸。（特别说明：沿前正中线向下触摸，找出胸骨体与剑突间形成的凹陷，该凹陷与肚脐连线的中点即为本穴。）

主要作用　治疗胃痛、胃胀、干呕、吞酸水等消化系统病症，对目眩、耳鸣、青春痘、精神差、神经衰弱也很有效。

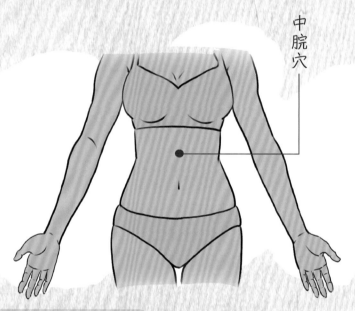

中脘穴

操作方法

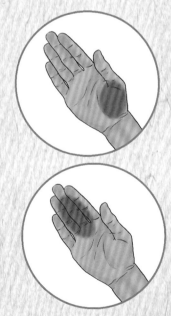

　　按揉，或艾条灸、隔姜灸。可用右手大鱼际，或四指并拢以中指为中心按揉中脘穴，一般顺时针按揉100次左右。对于有虚寒等虚性消化系统问题者或亚健康状态者，可以在中脘穴施以艾条灸或隔姜灸等。艾条温和灸或艾灸器灸时，局部有温热感、局部出现红晕即可，一般每次10～20分钟。隔姜灸，一般每次可以连续灸2～3壮。每周3次左右，灸后喝温开水。

Zhongwan Point (RN12)

Nomenclature   Middle means the point is between the Shangwan and Xiawan.

Location   On the anterior median line of the upper abdomen, 4.0 cun above the umbilicus. Or find the depression between sternum body and xiphoid process. Zhongwan is the middle point between the umbilicus and the depression.

Indications   Digestive disorders like epigastric pain, gastric distension, retching, acid regurgitation; vertigo, tinnitus, acne, low spirits, neurasthenia.

Methods   Press and rub Zhongwan point clockwise for 100 circles with the thenar eminence or the middle finger (with four fingers close to each other). Also, moxibustion can be used for 3 times a week to treat those with digestive diseases (deficiency) or sub-healthy problems. Hold a burning moxa stick above or place an apparatus with burning moxa sticks on Zhongwan point for 10 to 20 minutes until the area reddens. Or, ginger-partitioned moxibustion can be applied. 2 to 3 cones are needed in succession. Drink more warm water after moxibustion.

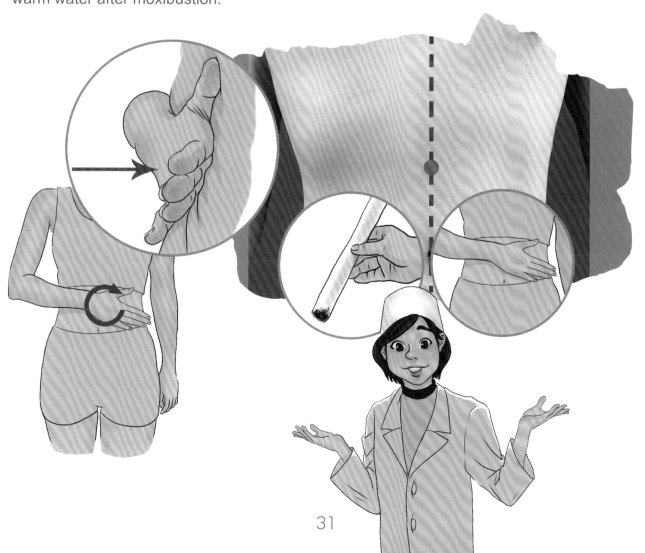

神阙穴

来　源　　神，神气；阙，原意为门楼、牌楼。神阙意指神气通行的门户。

位　置　　位于肚脐。

主要作用　　是人体生命最隐秘最关键的要害穴窍，是人体的长寿大穴。

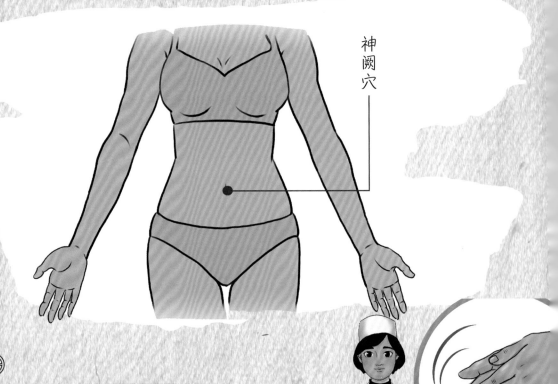

神阙穴

操作方法

　　每晚睡前空腹，将双手搓热，双手左下右上叠放于肚脐，顺时针揉转（女子相反），每次360下。也可以用艾灸的方法，如隔盐灸、隔姜灸、隔附子饼灸：首先在神阙穴上放置薄薄的一层相关隔物灸材料，而后在隔物灸材料上给予合适大小的艾绒艾炷施灸，每次2壮左右，施灸20分钟左右，每周2～3次。

Shenque Point (RN8)

Nomenclature Shen means spirit, while Que indicates archway. Shenque is an important passage for the circulation of the qi and spirit, like a palace gate of the spirit.

Location In the middle of the abdomen, in the center of the umbilicus.

Indications As a key point, Shenque can prolong the longevity.

Methods Tuina can be applied on an empty stomach at bedtime. Warm two hands by chafing and then rub the navel clockwise (anticlockwise for women) for 360 circles with left hand under the right one. Indirect moxibustion 2 to 3 times a week can also be useful. Keep a burning moxa cone at a certain distance from the skin with salt, ginger or aconite as insulating materials for 20 minutes. Two cones are needed.

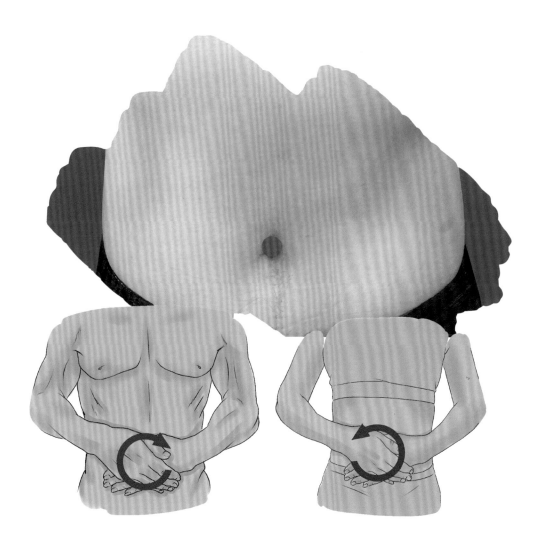

气海穴

来　源　意指任脉水气在此吸热后气化胀散，水气吸热胀散而化为充盛的天部之气，本穴如同气之海洋，故名气海。

位　置　位于腹正中线脐下1.5寸。

主要作用　治疗腹痛、腹泻、便秘等肠腑病症，夜尿症、阳痿、遗精、滑精、月经不调、闭经等妇科及泌尿生殖系统疾病，虚冷无力、精神差等气虚症状，以及脑血管病、气喘、心口窝疼、疝气、神经衰弱、儿童发育不良等。

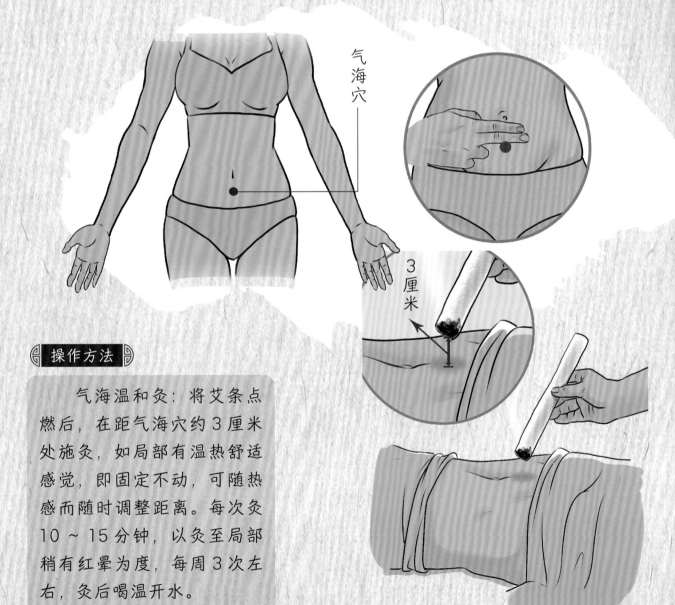

气海穴

3厘米

操作方法

　　气海温和灸：将艾条点燃后，在距气海穴约3厘米处施灸，如局部有温热舒适感觉，即固定不动，可随热感而随时调整距离。每次灸10～15分钟，以灸至局部稍有红晕为度，每周3次左右，灸后喝温开水。

Qihai Point (RN6)

Nomenclature   Water of Ren Meridian vaporizes here after being heated and forms into abundant heaven qi which makes the point a sea of qi.

Location   On the anterior median line of the lower abdomen, 1.5 cun below the umbilicus.

Indications   Intestinal diseases like abdominal pain, diarrhea, constipation; gynecological and reproductive disorders like nocturnal urination, impotence, spermatorrhea, irregular menstruation, amenorrhea; fatigue, flaccidity, cerebrovascular disease, asthma, cardiac pain, hernia, neurasthenia, dysplasia.

Methods   Moxibustion can be used for 3 times a week. Hold a burning moxa stick 3 centimeters above Qihai point for 10 to 15 minutes until the area reddens and becomes suffused with warmth. The distance between the point and the moxa stick can be adjusted according to the heat sensation. Drink more warm water after moxibustion.

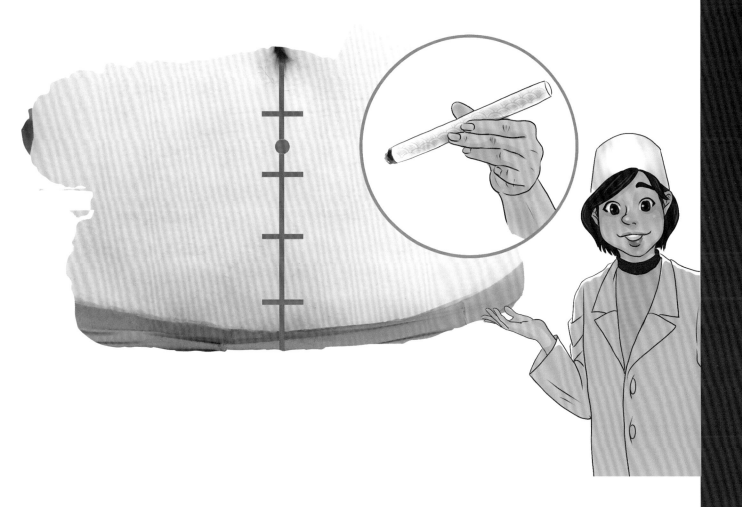

关元穴

来　源
为先天之气海，是养生吐纳吸气凝神的地方，古人称之为人身元阴元阳交关之处，是足太阴经、足少阴经、足厥阴经与任脉的交会穴。

位　置
位于脐下 3 寸处。

主要作用
用于治疗阳痿、早泄、遗精、尿频等泌尿生殖系统疾患，痛经、白带异常、月经不调等妇科病，腹痛、腹泻、脱肛等肠腑病症，以及怕冷无力、精神差等症状。

操作方法

　　艾条灸、艾灸器灸或者隔姜灸。艾条温和灸时要离皮肤适当距离，一般 3～5 厘米，局部有温热感即可，避免烫伤。艾灸器有各种艾灸盒，将艾条按要求放入艾灸盒内点燃施灸，方便安全，效果以局部出现红晕、温暖舒适即可，一般每次 10～20 分钟。隔姜灸时姜片厚度取 3 毫米左右，直径 3 厘米左右即可，将艾绒搓成小艾炷放置在姜片上施灸，艾绒熄灭才能取下，内科疾病一般每次可以连续灸 2～3 壮。每周 3 次左右，灸后喝温开水。

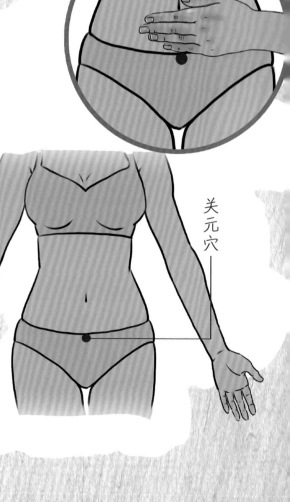

关元穴

Guanyuan Point (RN4)

Nomenclature   As a congenital sea of qi, Guanyuan is a storage place for the primary qi of the body and spirit. It is the place where Foot-Taiyin, Foot-Shaoyin, Foot-Jueyin Meridians and Ren Meridian cross.

Location   On the anterior median line of the lower abdomen, 3 cun below the umbilicus.

Indications   Reproductive and urinary disorders like impotence, premature ejaculation, spermatorrhea and frequent micturition; gynecological diseases like dysmenorrhea, morbid leukorrhea, and irregular menstruation; intestinal diseases like abdominal pain, diarrhea and prolapse of rectum; other symptoms like aversion to cold, fatigue and flaccidity.

Methods   Moxibustion can be used for 3 times a week. Hold a burning moxa stick 3 to 5 centimeters above the surface of the skin until the area reddens and becomes suffused with warmth. Or, put burning moxa sticks in the moxibustion apparatus and place the apparatus on the point for 10 to 20 minutes until the area become flushed. Or, keep a burning moxa cone on a 3-mm-thick ginger slice (3-cm diameter) until the burning cone dies out. To treat internal disorders, 2 to 3 cones are needed. Drink more warm water after moxibustion.

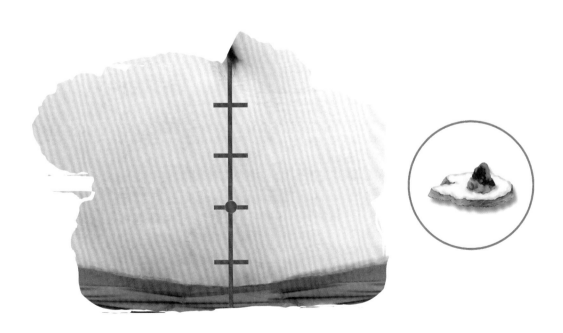

中极穴

来　源　意指任脉气血在此达到了天部中的最高点。本穴物质为曲骨穴传来的阴湿水气，其上升至中极时已达到其所能上升的最高点。

位　置　位于人体前正中线，脐下4寸。

主要作用　治疗生殖系统疾病，泌尿系统疾病如尿频、尿急，精力差，冷感症等。此穴位为人体任脉上的主要穴位之一。

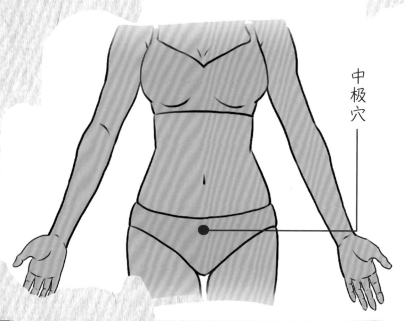

中极穴

操作方法

艾条灸、艾灸器灸或者隔姜灸。艾条温和灸时要离皮肤适当距离，一般为3～5厘米，局部有温热感即可，注意不要烫伤。艾灸器有各种艾灸盒，将艾条按要求放入艾灸盒内点燃施灸，方便安全，效果以局部出现红晕、温暖舒适即可，一般每次10～20分钟。隔姜灸时姜片厚度取3毫米左右，直径3厘米左右即可，将艾绒搓成小艾炷放置在姜片上施灸，艾绒熄灭才能取下，内科疾病一般每次可以连续灸2～3壮。每周3次左右，灸后喝温开水。

Zhongji Point (RN3)

Nomenclature Zhongji is the highest point where qi and blood of Ren Meridian (damp water flowing from Qugu point) can reach.

Location On the anterior median line of the lower abdomen, 4 cun below the umbilicus.

Indications As a main point in Ren Meridian, it can be used to treat reproductive disorders, urinary diseases like frequent micturition, urgent urination, fatigue and cold sensation.

Methods Moxibustion can be used for 3 times a week. Hold a burning moxa stick 3 to 5 centimeters above the surface of the skin until the area reddens and becomes suffused with warmth. Or, put burning moxa sticks in the moxibustion apparatus and place the apparatus on the point for 10 to 20 minutes until the area become flushed. Or, keep a burning moxa cone on a 3-mm-thick ginger slice (3-cm diameter) until the burning cone dies out. To treat internal disorders, 2 to 3 cones are needed. Drink more warm water after moxibustion.

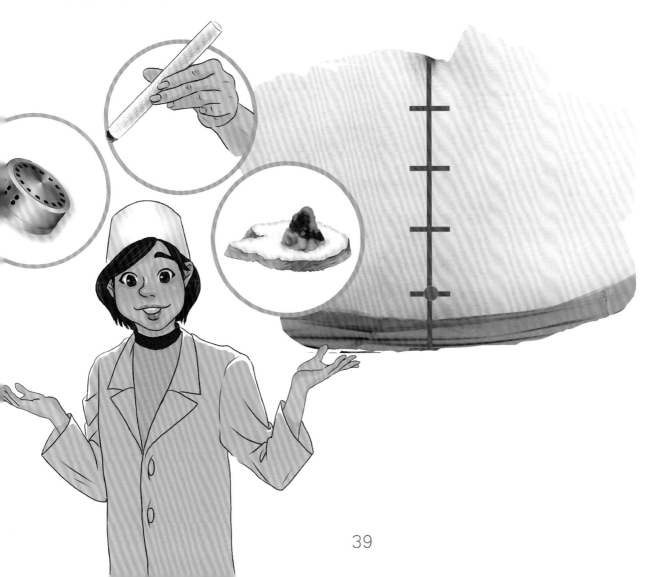

天枢穴

来　源　　上走与胃经处于相近层次的大肠经，也就是向更高的天部输送，故名天枢。

位　置　　脐中旁开 2 寸。仰卧，人体中腹部，肚脐向左右旁开 2 寸处。

主要作用　　临床常用穴位，其应用以治疗肠胃疾病为主。经临床研究发现，天枢穴有其特殊的作用，对肠腑功能异常有明显的双向性调节作用，既能治疗腹泻，又能治疗便秘。

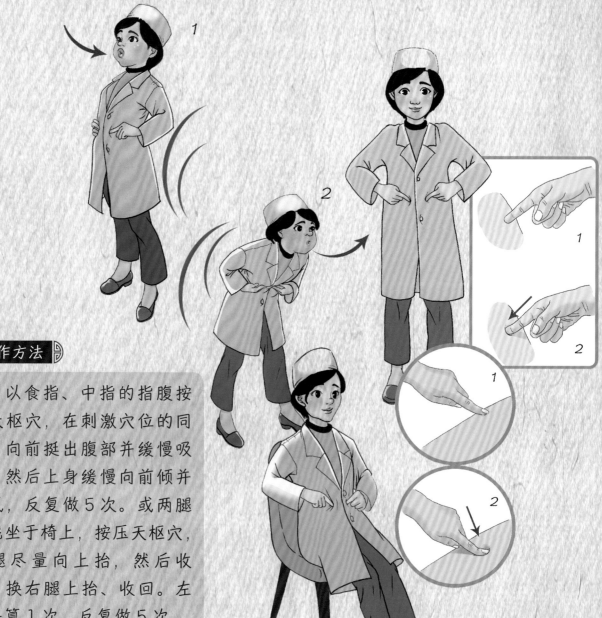

操作方法

以食指、中指的指腹按压天枢穴，在刺激穴位的同时，向前挺出腹部并缓慢吸气，然后上身缓慢向前倾并呼气，反复做 5 次。或两腿并拢坐于椅上，按压天枢穴，左腿尽量向上抬，然后收回；换右腿上抬、收回。左右共算 1 次，反复做 5 次。

40

Tianshu Point (ST25)

Nomenclature   Qi and blood of Tianshu point goes upwards to Large Intestine Meridian which pertains to heaven.

Location   On the middle of the abdomen, 2 cun lateral to the umbilicus.

Indications   Tianshu is a main point to treat gastrointestinal diseases. It is found that Tianshu has its special effect on regulating the intestines. It can treat not only diarrhea, but also constipation.

Methods   Press Tianshu with the pulp of index finger and middle finger when inhaling gradually and expanding the belly. Next, lean forward slowly and exhale. Repeat it for 5 times. Or, sit on the chair with no space between the two legs. Next press Tianshu while taking turns raising the left leg and then the right leg as high as possible. Repeat it for 5 times.

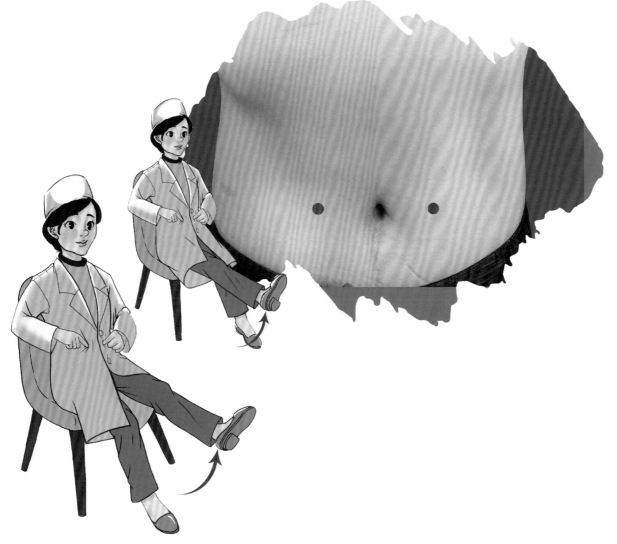

41

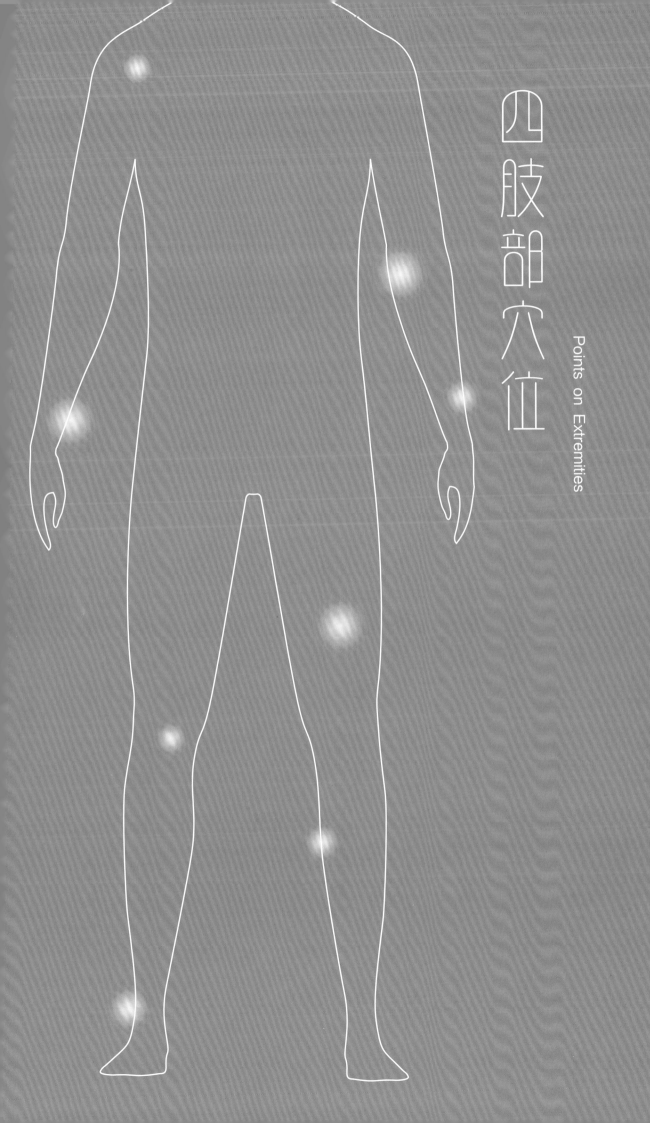

四肢部穴位

Points on Extremities

合谷穴

| 来　源 | 意指大肠经气血汇聚于此并形成强盛的水湿风气场。 |

位　置　　在手背，第1、第2掌骨之间，当第2掌骨桡侧之中点处。（特别说明：伸臂，拇指食指张开，以一手的拇指指间横纹放在另一手拇指食指指间的指蹼缘上，屈指，拇指尖所指处，按压有明显酸胀感，即为本穴。）

主要作用　　《四总穴歌》说："面口合谷收。"本穴位是治疗热病发热及头面五官各种疾患之要穴，如头痛、目赤肿痛、牙痛，无汗、多汗，以及急性腰扭伤、落枕、腕关节痛、膈肌痉挛等其他内外科疾病。

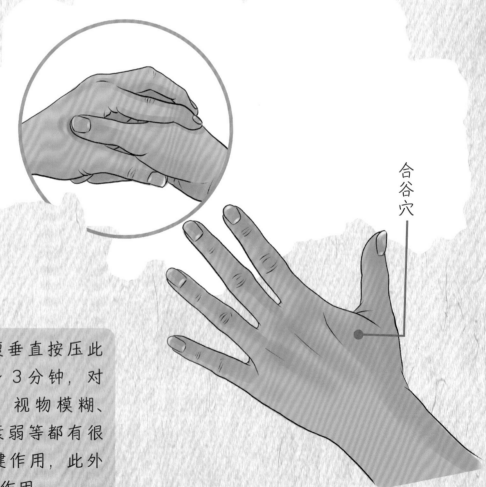

合谷穴

操作方法

拇指指腹垂直按压此穴，每次1~3分钟，对头痛、耳聋、视物模糊、失眠、神经衰弱等都有很好的调理保健作用，此外还有健脾胃的作用。

Hegu Point (LI4)

Nomenclature The qi and blood of large intestines accumulates here and forms into a valley where is filled with water, dampness and wind.

Location On the dorsum of the hand, between the 1st and 2nd metacarpal bones, in the middle of the 2nd metacarpal bone on the radial side. Or, place the transverse crease of the interphalangeal joint of the thumb against the web margin between the thumb and the index finger of the other hand. The point is where the tip of the thumb touches.

Indications This is the main point for diseases of the head and face, fever and febrile diseases. For example, headache, swelling and pain of the eye, toothache; anhidrosis, hidrosis; acute waist sprain, stiff neck, wrist pain; phrenospasm.

Methods Press the point perpendicularly with the pulp of the thumb for 1 to 3 minutes. It can treat deafness, blurred vision, insomnia and neurasthenia. It can strengthen spleen and stomach as well.

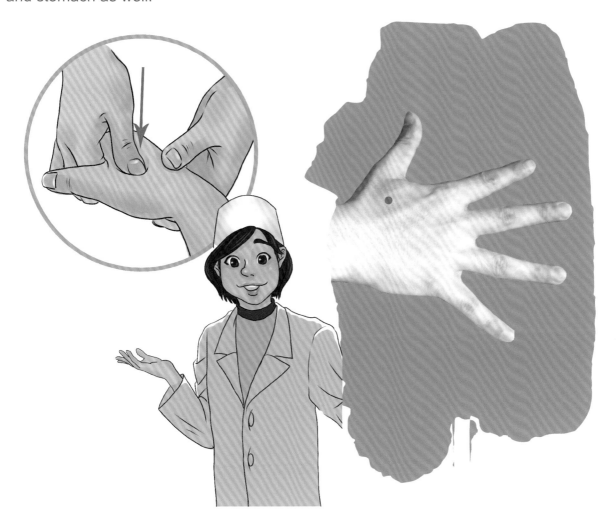

鱼际穴

来　源　拇指对掌肌边缘处肌肉丰隆，形如鱼腹，此穴又当赤白肉际相会之处，故名。

位　置　第1掌指关节后，第1掌骨中点，掌后白肉隆起（大鱼际肌）的边缘（赤白肉际），按压有酸胀处，即为本穴。

主要作用　主治咽干、咽喉肿痛、声音嘶哑、咳嗽、咯血，小儿头发稀疏、干枯无光，多汗症，鼻出血，乳腺炎，手指肿痛。

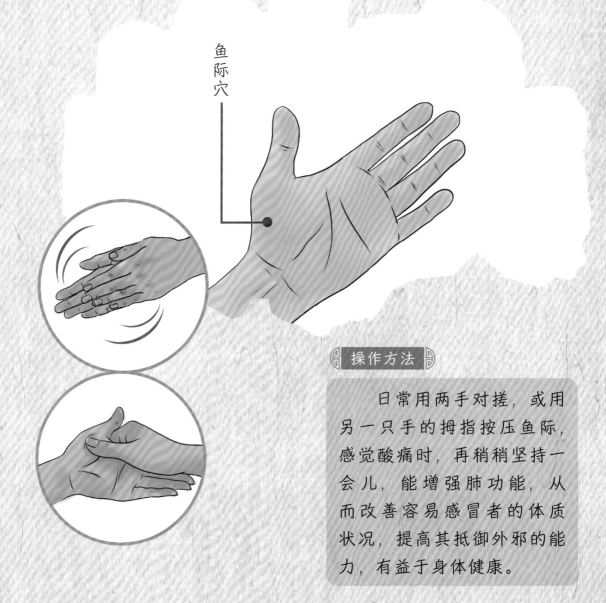

鱼际穴

操作方法

　　日常用两手对搓，或用另一只手的拇指按压鱼际，感觉酸痛时，再稍稍坚持一会儿，能增强肺功能，从而改善容易感冒者的体质状况，提高其抵御外邪的能力，有益于身体健康。

Yuji Point (LU10)

Nomenclature The musculi flexor pollicis in the palm are prominent like a fish, the point is located just on its border.

Location On the margin behind the thenar eminence of the thumb, about the midpoint of the radial side of the first metacarpal bone, on the junction of the red and white skin.

Indications Dry or sore throat, hoarseness, cough, hemoptysis (coughing blood), thinning and lackluster hair of kids, hyperhidrosis, nose bleeding, mastitis, sore fingers.

Methods Rub two hands. Or keep pressing Yuji point with the thumb until you feel sore for a while, which can strengthen lung functions, improve immunity, prevent common cold and keep healthy.

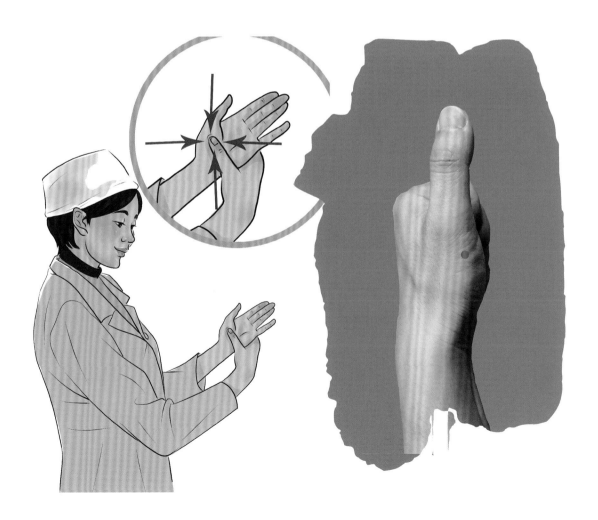

47

落枕穴

来　源	是治疗睡觉时落枕的特效穴位，因而被命名为落枕穴。

位　置	位于手背侧，当第 2、第 3 掌骨之间，掌指关节后约 0.5 寸处。

主要作用	治疗落枕、手臂痛、胃痛。

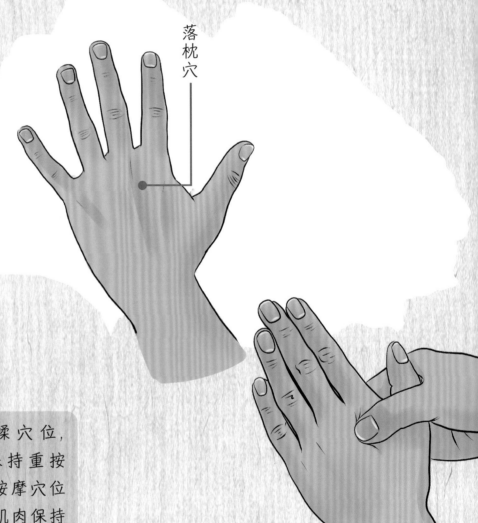

落枕穴

操作方法

以大拇指按揉穴位，用力由轻到重，保持重按 10 ～ 15 分钟，在按摩穴位的过程中，使颈部肌肉保持松弛，将头轻轻缓慢地左右转动，幅度由小逐渐加大，并将颈部逐渐伸直到正常位置。

Laozhen Point (EX-UE8)

Nomenclature It's a point with special effects in treating stiff neck due to sleep posture.

Location On the dorsal side of the hand between the 2nd and 3rd metacarpal bones, about 0.5 cun behind the metacarpal and phalangeal joints.

Indications Stiff neck, arm pain, stomachache.

Methods Press and rub the point with thumb first gently and then forcefully for 10 to 15 minutes. When rubbing the point, relax the muscles of the neck and gently turn the head until the neck can reach the normal position.

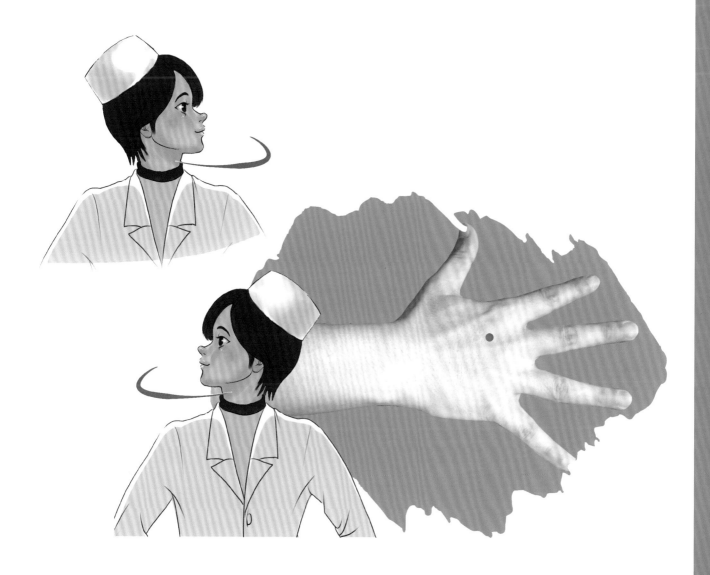

列缺穴

来　源　　此穴为手太阴肺经之络穴，络脉自此分出别走手阳明大肠经。位于桡骨茎突上方，当肱桡肌腱与拇长展肌腱之间，有如裂隙处，故名。

位　置　　在前臂桡侧缘，桡骨茎突上方，腕横纹上1.5寸。[特别说明：两虎口相交，一手食指压在另一手桡骨茎突（掌心向前，手腕外侧突起的骨头）上，在食指尖端到达的凹陷处，触摸时可感有一裂隙，即为本穴。]

主要作用　　《四总穴歌》："头项寻列缺。"本穴位对于偏头痛、颈项僵痛、三叉神经痛、健忘、胆小易惊等病症，可以起到显著的保健调理效果。

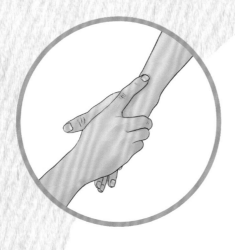

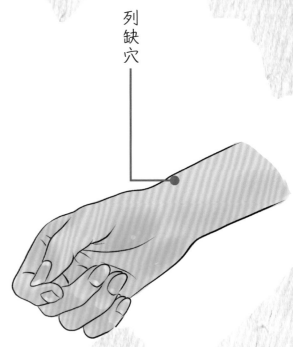

列缺穴

操作方法

　　每天坚持用食指指腹揉按列缺，每次1～3分钟。

Lieque Point (LU7)

Nomenclature   The Hand-Taiyin Meridian branches from this point to connect the Hand-Yangming Meridian. The point is in the depression superior to the styloid process of the radius.

Location   On the radial margin of the forearm, superior to the styloid process of the radius,1.5 cun above the transverse crease of the wrist. Or, place the web margin between the thumb and the index finger against the web margin between the thumb and the index finger of the other hand, then put the index finger on the styloid process of the radius. The point is between the two tendons where the tip of the index finger touches.

Indications   It is an effective point for migraine, stiff neck, neck pain, trigeminal neuralgia, forgetfulness and timidity.

Methods   Rub Lieque with the pulp of index finger for 1 to 3 minutes everyday.

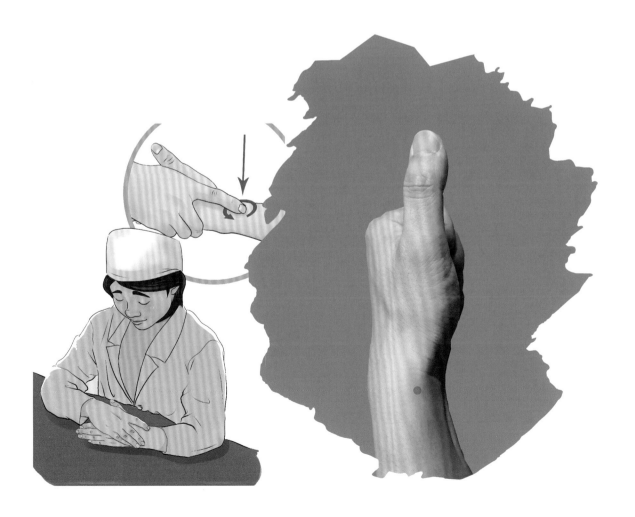

外关穴

| 来　源 | 意指三焦经气血在此胀散外行，外部气血被关卡不得入于三焦经，故名。 |

| 位　置 | 腕背横纹上2寸，尺骨与桡骨之间。（特别说明：与内关穴相对。） |

| 主要作用 | 治疗手指疼痛、手臂屈伸困难、头痛、眼睛红肿、耳鸣、耳聋、胸胁痛等。 |

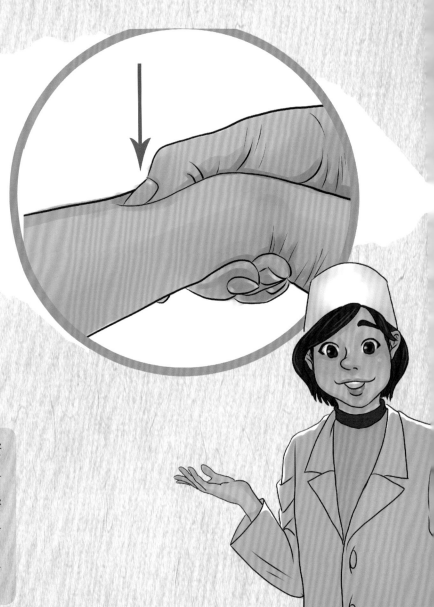

| 操作方法 |

　　用左手的拇指指尖按压在右侧外关穴上，左手食指压在右侧内关上，按捏10～15分钟，再用右手按压左侧的穴位，反复操作即可。每日2～3次。

Waiguan Point (SJ5)

Nomenclature   Qi and blood of Sanjiao Meridian disperses at this point and the point works as a pass and prevent the external qi and blood from flowing into Sanjiao Meridian.

Location   2 cun above the transverse crease of the wrist between the ulna and radius. The point is opposite to Neiguan point which is located on the inside of the arm.

Indications   Finger pain, difficulty in flexion and extension of arms, headache, red and swollen eyes, tinnitus, deafness, pain in the hypochondrium.

Methods   Press Waiguan point with the tip of the thumb and Neiguan point with the index finger for 2 to 3 times a day with 10 to 15 minutes each time.

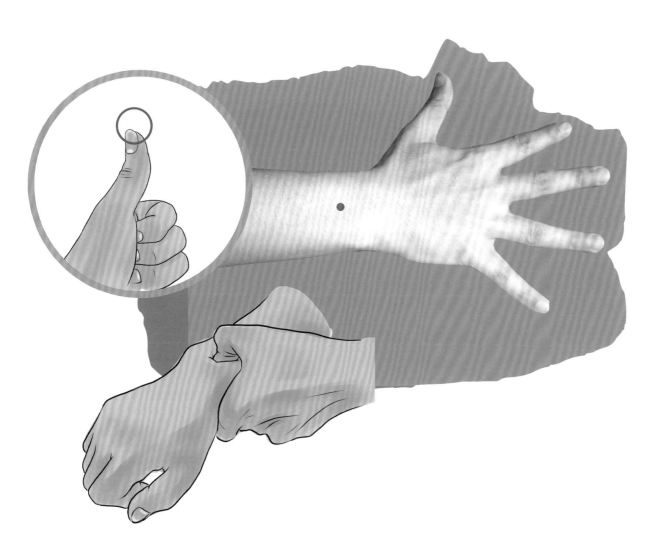

支沟穴

来源 意指三焦经气血在此吸热扩散，此气按其自身的阳热特性循三焦经经脉渠道向上、向外而行，扩散之气亦如树之分叉，故名。

位置 在前臂背侧，当腕背横纹中央凹陷与肘尖的连线上，腕背横纹上3寸。

主要作用 《四总穴歌》："胸胁支沟取。"本穴可治疗便秘、胁肋痛、耳鸣、耳聋、咽痛声哑、腰痛等。

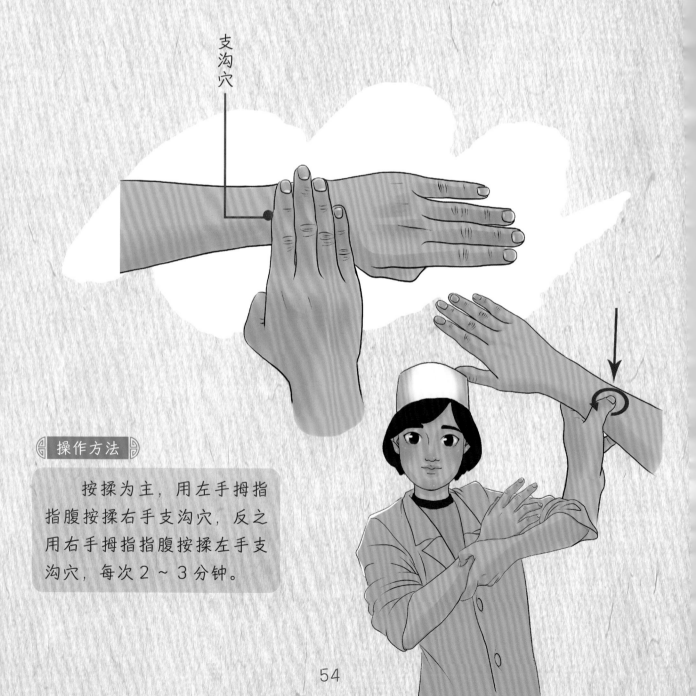

支沟穴

操作方法

按揉为主，用左手拇指指腹按揉右手支沟穴，反之用右手拇指指腹按揉左手支沟穴，每次2～3分钟。

Zhigou Point (SJ6)

Nomenclature Qi and blood of Sanjiao Meridian disperses upwards and outwards at this point after being heated like branches.

Location On the dorsal aspect of the forearm, on the line connecting SJ4 and the tip of the elbow, 3 cun above the transverse crease of the wrist between the ulna and radius.

Indications Constipation, pain in the hypochondrium, tinnitus, deafness, sore throat, hoarseness, lumbar pain.

Methods Press and rub Zhigou with the pulp of the thumb for 2 to 3 minutes.

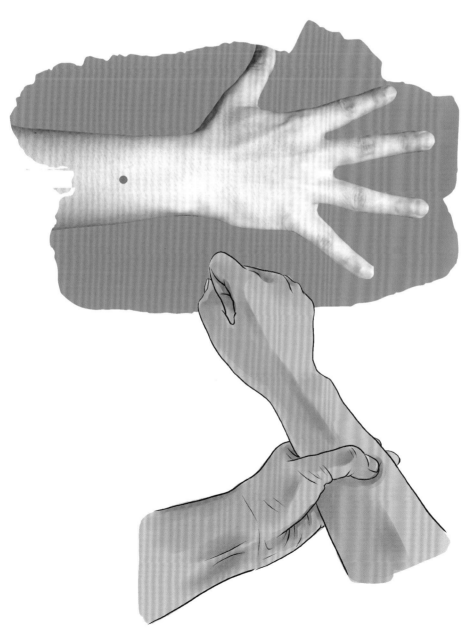

曲池穴

来　源　脉气流注此穴时，似水注入池中；又取穴时，屈曲其肘，横纹头有凹陷，形似浅池。故名曲池。

位　置　屈肘成45°，在肘关节的外侧，肘横纹头处，即为本穴，当尺泽与肱骨外上髁连线中点。

主要作用　主治手臂痹痛、上肢不遂等上肢病症，热病，高血压，腹痛、吐泻等胃肠病，咽喉肿痛、牙痛等五官病症，瘾疹、湿疹、颈部淋巴结肿大等皮肤外科疾病。

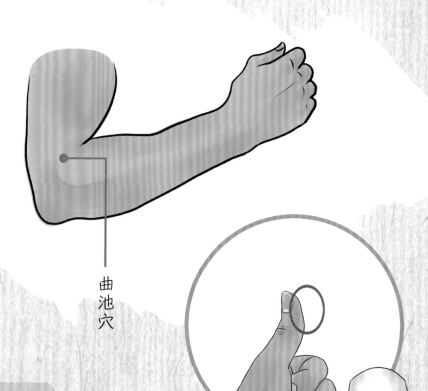

曲池穴

操作方法

每天早晚用拇指指腹垂直按压曲池，每次1～3分钟，可改善上肢瘫麻、哮喘等；每日按压曲池穴1～2分钟，使酸胀感向下扩散，有预防高血压的作用。

Quchi Point (LI11)

Nomenclature Qi flows into this point as if water flows into a pool. The point is located on the depression at the elbow like a pool when the arm is bent and this point is inside it.

Location With the elbow flexed, the point is on the lateral end of the transverse cubital crease, at midpoint between LU5 and the lateral epicondyle of the humerus.

Indications Problems of upper limbs like arm pain and stiffness; all febrile diseases; hypertension; gastrointestinal diseases like abdominal pain, vomiting and diarrhea; disorders of five sense organs like sore throat, toothache; skin problems like urticaria, eczema and enlargement of cervical lymph nodes.

Methods Press Quchi perpendicularly with the pulp of the thumb for 1 to 3 minutes to improve numbness and paralysis in upper limbs and asthma. To prevent hypertension, press this point for 1 to 2 minutes each day until a sensation of soreness goes downwards.

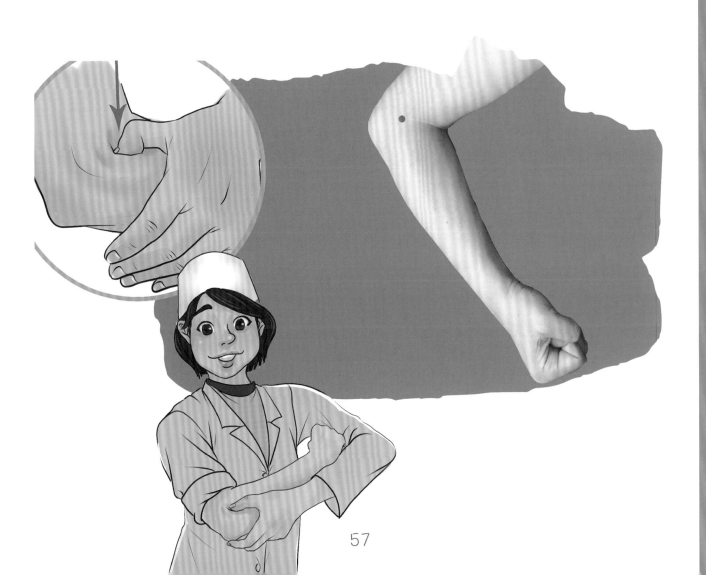

内关穴

| 来　源 | 意指心包经的体表经水由此注入体内，其气化之气无法从本穴的地部孔隙外出体表，如被关卡阻挡一般，故而本穴得名内关。 |

| 位　置 | 位于前臂掌侧，当曲泽与大陵的连线上，腕横纹上2寸、掌长肌腱与桡侧腕屈肌腱之间。（特别说明：伸臂，手掌向上，微屈拳。在手臂的内侧可以看到明显的两条大筋，从靠近手腕横纹的地方向上量2寸，两筋之间的凹陷处，即为本穴。） |

| 主要作用 | 内关为常用特定穴，亦是全身强壮要穴之一，《四总穴歌》："心胸内关谋。"本穴可治疗心绞痛、心肌炎、心律不齐、胃炎、晕车、恶心等。 |

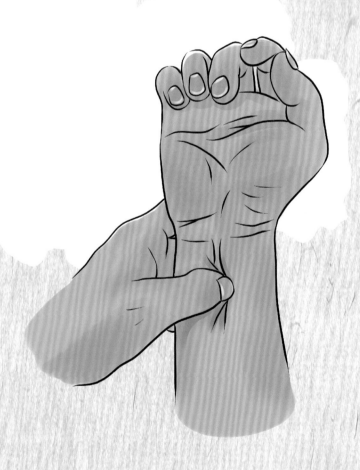

| 操作方法 | 用左手的拇指指尖按压在右侧内关穴上，左手食指压在右侧外关上，按捏10～15分钟，再用右手按压左侧的穴位，反复操作即可。每日2～3次。 |

Neiguan Point (PC6)

Nomenclature   Water of Pericardium Meridian on the body surface flows into the inside body at this point. The point works as a pass and prevent inside qi flowing out.

Location   On the palmar aspect of the forearm, 2 cun above the transverse crease of the wrist, on the line connecting PC3 and PC7, between the tendons of palmaris longus and fexor carpi radialis. Make a fist slightly with the palm up and two tendons will be easily found on the palmar aspect of the arm. The point is 2 cun above the transverse crease between the two tendons.

Indications   As a key point with special effects, Neiguan point is responsible for angina, myocarditis, arrhythmia, gastritis, carsickness, nausea and so on.

Methods   Press Neiguan point with the tip of the thumb and Waiguan point with the index finger for 2 to 3 times a day with 10 to 15 minutes each time.

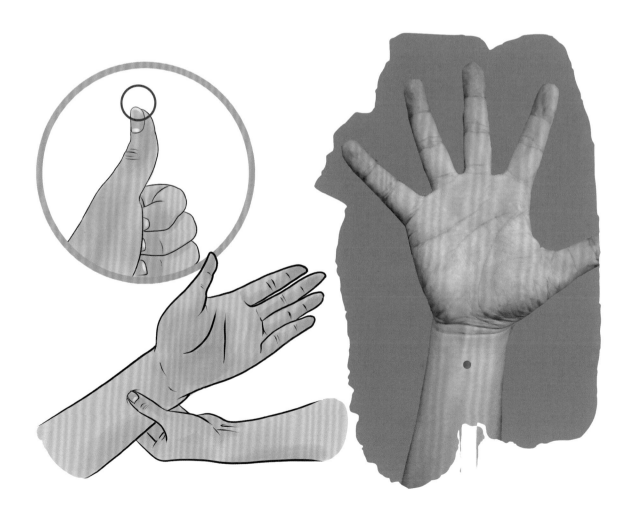

神门穴

来　源　　意指心经体内经脉的气血物质由此交于心经体表经脉。其气性同心经气血之本性，为人之神气，故名神门。

位　置　　位于腕部，腕掌侧横纹尺侧端，尺侧腕屈肌腱的桡侧凹陷处。（特别说明：取穴时伸开手臂，握紧拳头，在手臂内侧面可以摸到一条大筋，在靠近手腕横纹的地方，此筋的内侧即为本穴。）

主要作用　　为安神要穴，主治心病，包括心烦、胸闷、心慌、健忘、失眠、胸胁痛等。

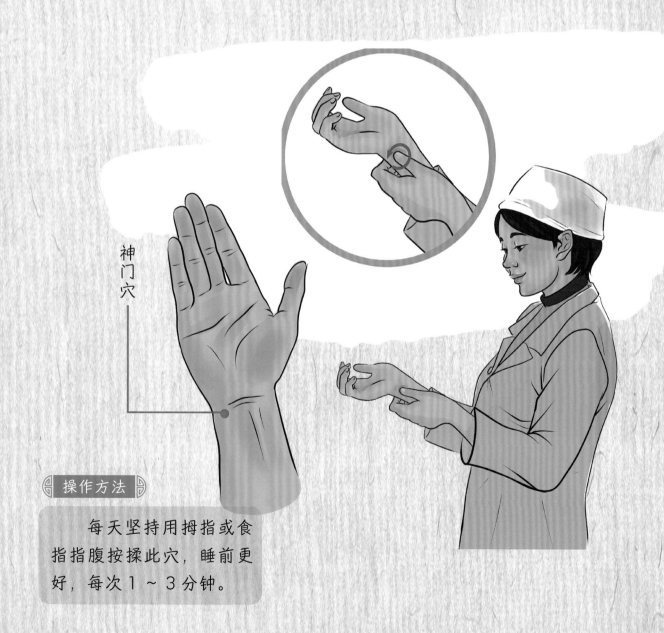

神门穴

操作方法

　　每天坚持用拇指或食指指腹按揉此穴，睡前更好，每次1～3分钟。

Shenmen Point (HT7)

Nomenclature Qi and blood of the inside part of Heart Meridian flows to this point and joins to the part on the body surface. The heart houses the mind. This point is a door for the mind.

Location On the wrist, at the ulnar end of the transverse crease of the wrist, in the depression on the radial side of the tendon of flexor carpi ulnaris. Make a fist firmly and you will feel a large tendon at the ulnar end of the transverse crease of the wrist. The point is on the radial side of the tendon.

Indications As a key point for tranquilization, Shenmen can treat cardiac disorders, including anxiety, chest tightness, palpitation, forgetfulness, insomnia, chest pain and so on.

Methods Keep pressing and rubbing Shenmen point with the pulp of thumb or index finger for 1 to 3 minutes every day. It's better to do it before sleep.

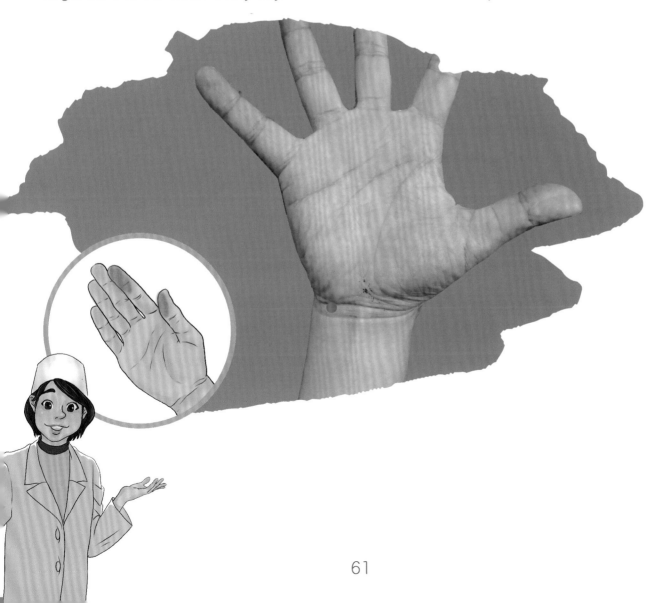

劳宫穴

| 来　源 | 因"手任劳作，穴在掌心"而定名为劳宫穴。 |

| 位　置 | 位于手掌心，当第 2、第 3 掌骨之间偏于第 3 掌骨，握拳屈指时中指尖处。 |

| 主要作用 | 是清心火的要穴，可治疗昏迷、中暑、癔病、口腔炎等。 |

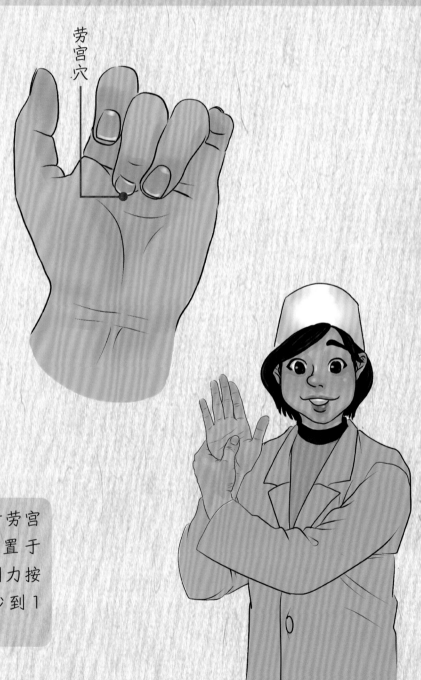

劳宫穴

操作方法

拇指按压于劳宫穴，其余四指置于手背处，拇指用力按压揉动约 30 秒到 1 分钟。

Laogong Point (PC8)

Nomenclature   The hand is used for labour. Laogong is in the centre of the palm.

Location   In the center of the palm, between the 2nd and 3rd metacarpal bones, closer to the 3rd metacarpal bone. When a fist is made, the point is where the tip of the middle finger touches.

Indications   Laogong point, as a key point to clear Heart-Fire, can treat coma, heat stroke, hysteria, stomatitis.

Methods   Press and rub Laogong point with the thumb (the other four fingers placing on the back of the palm) for 30 to 60 seconds.

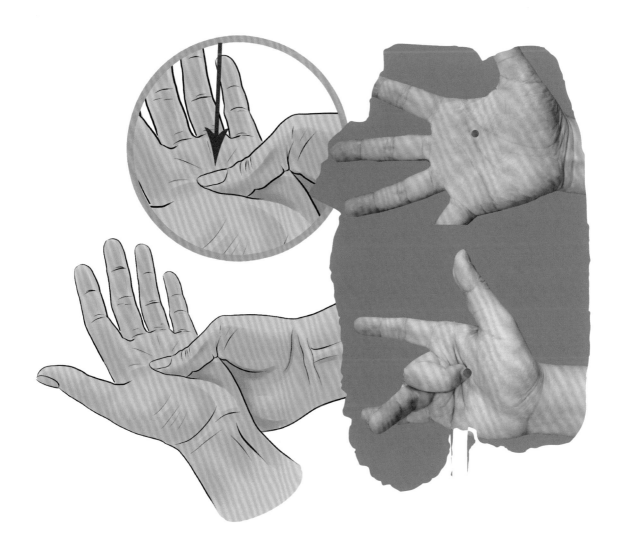

风市穴

来　源　　意指胆经经气在此散热冷缩后化为水湿风气，如同风气的集散之地。

位　置　　直立，手下垂于体侧，中指尖所到处即是。

主要作用　　常用于治疗皮肤瘙痒、头痛、眩晕、坐骨神经痛、股外侧皮神经炎。

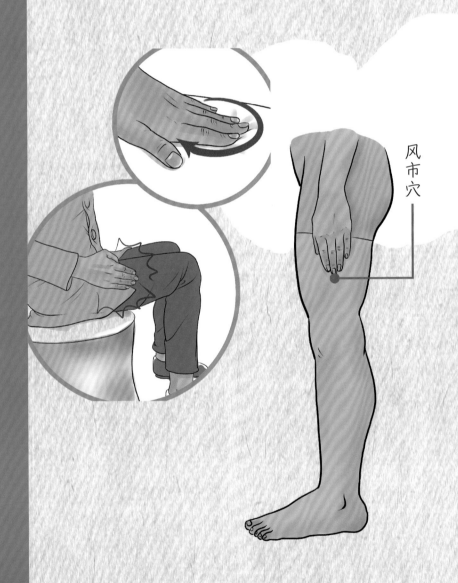

风市穴

操作方法

　　按揉或拍打，用同侧手四指并拢，以中指指腹按揉大腿外侧风市穴，或者用同侧并拢的手指拍打，每次2～3分钟。也可以用艾灸温和灸的方法祛风散寒。

Fengshi Point (GB31)

Nomenclature Qi of Gallbladder Meridian disperses here and transforms into damp wind qi after encountering cold. This point is like a market gathering wind and qi.

Location On the midline of the lateral aspect of the thigh, 7 cun above the transverse popliteal crease. When the patient is standing erect with the hands hanging down close to the sides, the point is where the tip of the middle finger touches.

Indications Skin pruritus, headache, vertigo, sciatica, lateral femoral cutaneous neuritis.

Methods Press or rub Fengshi with the pulp of middle finger (four fingers close to each other) for 2 to 3 minutes. Or, pat the point with four fingers together for 2 to 3 minutes. Moxibustion is also effective in expelling wind and cold.

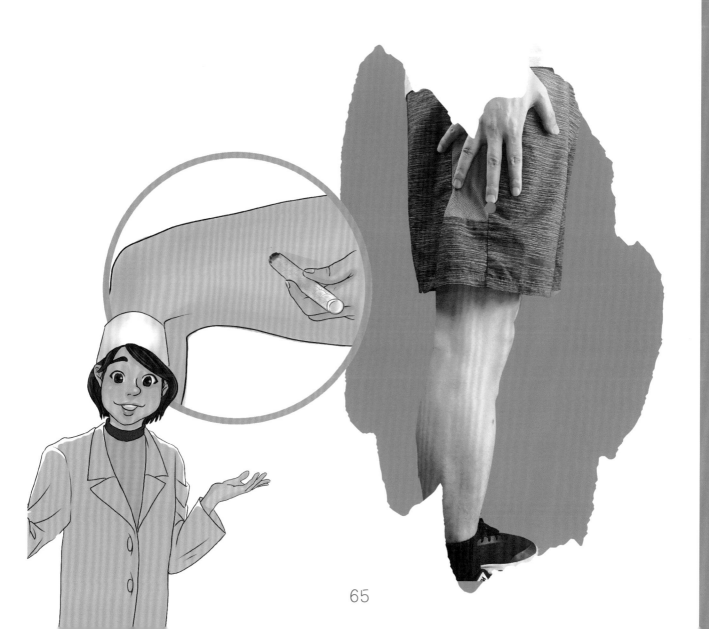

65

委中穴

| 来 源 | 意指膀胱经的湿热水气在此为聚集之状，故名委中。 |

| 位 置 | 位于人体的腘横纹中点，当左右两大筋（股二头肌腱与半腱肌肌腱）的中间。 |

| 主要作用 | 《四总穴歌》："腰背委中求。" 本穴可用于治疗急性胃肠炎、中暑、腰背痛、足挛痛、急性腰扭伤等。 |

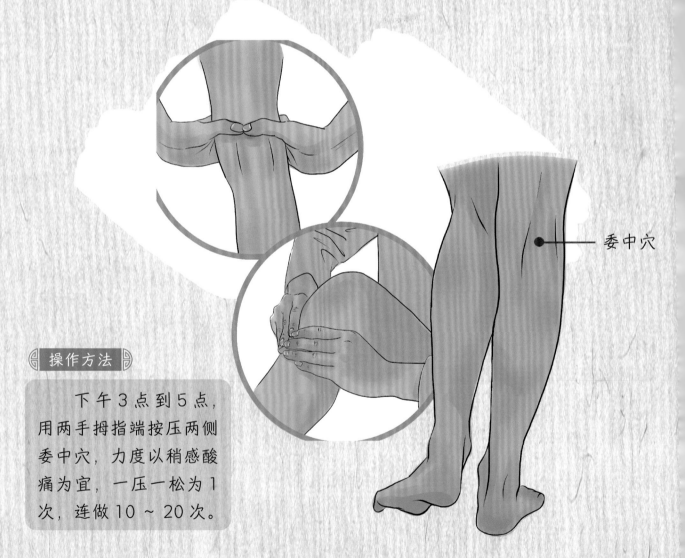

委中穴

操作方法

下午3点到5点，用两手拇指端按压两侧委中穴，力度以稍感酸痛为宜，一压一松为1次，连做10～20次。

Weizhong Point (BL40)

Nomenclature   Dampness and heat of Bladder Meridian accumulates at the midpoint of the transverse crease of the popliteal fossa.

Location   Midpoint of the transverse crease of the popliteal fossa, between the tendons of biceps femoris and semitendinosus.

Indications   Acute gastroenteritis, heat stroke, lumbar back pain, foot pain, acute lumbar sprain.

Methods   Choose to have tuina at 3 to 5 o'clock in the afternoon. Press Weizhong points with thumbs until you feel slightly sore and then release. Repeat it for 10 to 20 times.

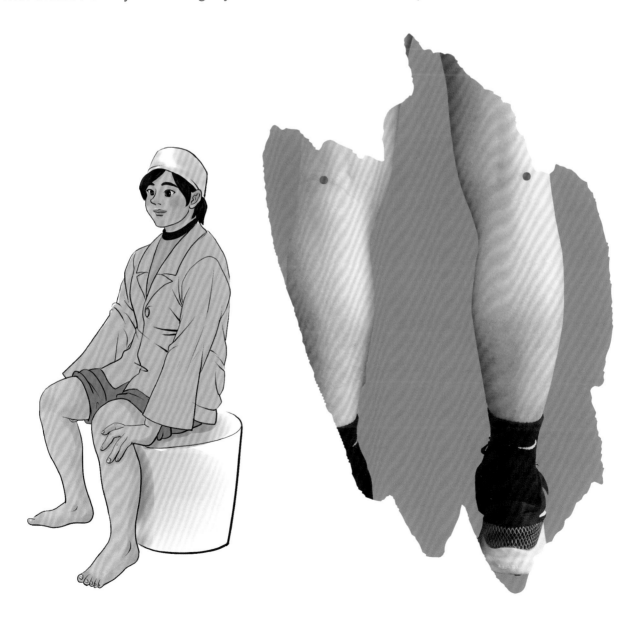

足三里穴

来　源　因本穴在膝下 3 寸，所以称足三里，是胃的下合穴。

位　置　由外膝眼向下量 4 横指，在腓骨与胫骨之间，由胫骨旁量 1 横指（中指）。

主要作用　为全身强壮要穴之一，能调节改善机体免疫功能，有防病保健作用。《四总穴歌》中说："肚腹三里留。"常用于治疗腹部疾病，如胃痛、呕吐、腹胀、腹泻、便秘、消化不良，以及心律失常、失眠等。

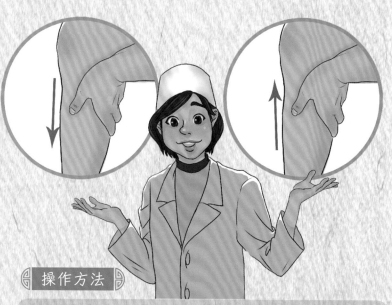

操作方法

胃胀、胃脘疼痛的时候就要"理上"，按足三里的时候要同时往上方使劲；腹部正中出现不适，就需要"理中"，只用往内按就行了；小腹在肚腹的下部，小腹上的病痛，得在按住足三里的同时往下方使劲，这叫"理下"。对足三里施灸时，取清艾条 1 根，将其点燃后靠近足三里熏烤，艾条距穴位约 3 厘米，如局部有温热舒适感觉，就固定不动，每次灸 10 ~ 15 分钟，以灸至局部稍有红晕为度，隔日可以施灸 1 次，每月总共灸 10 次即可。

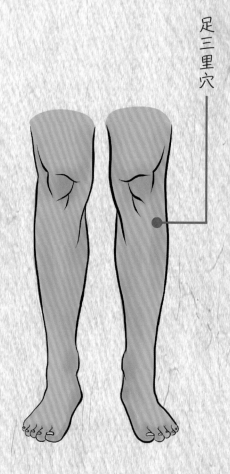

足三里穴

Zusanli Point (ST36)

Nomenclature Zusanli is on the leg, 3 cun below the knee.

Location On the anterior aspect of the lower leg, 3 cun below ST 35, one finger-breadth (middle finger) from the anterior crest of the tibia.

Indications As a main point for strengthening the body and improving immunity, it can treat abdominal disorders, such as gastric pain, vomiting, abdominal distention, diarrhea, constipation and indigestion. Arrhythmia and insomnia are also indications.

Methods Press Zusanli upwards when treating stomach distension and pain; press it inwards when treating abdominal discomfort; press it downwards when treating problems in lower abdomen. Or, hold a burning moxa stick 3 centimeters away from the point for 10 to 15 minutes until the area reddens. Moxibustion can be applied every other day, for 10 times per month in total.

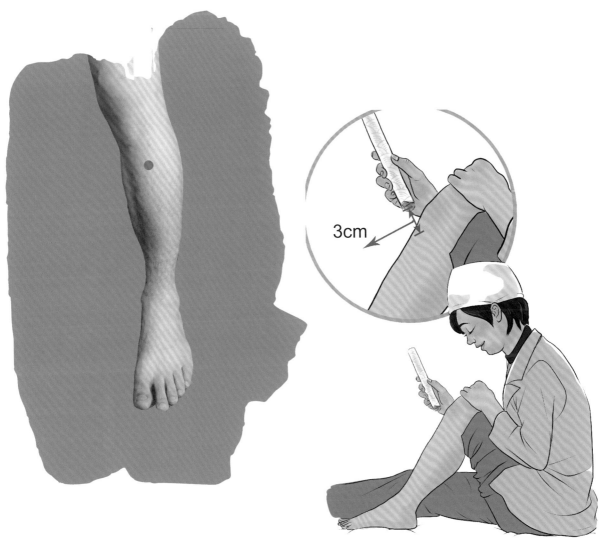

3cm

阴陵泉穴

来　源　　本穴在胫骨内侧髁下缘凹陷中，如山陵下之水泉，故名阴陵泉。

位　置　　位于小腿内侧，胫骨内侧髁下缘与胫骨内侧缘之间的凹陷中。

主要作用　　是健脾利水的要穴，治疗急慢性肠炎、细菌性痢疾、尿潴留、尿失禁、尿路感染、阴道炎、下肢水肿、膝关节及周围软组织疾患。

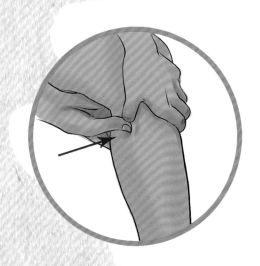

阴陵泉穴

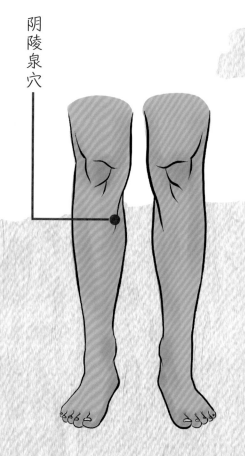

操作方法

　　拇指指端放于阴陵泉穴处，先顺时针方向按揉2分钟，再点按半分钟，以酸胀为度。艾灸也可以，温和灸操作见前述穴位。

Yinlingquan Point (SP9)

Nomenclature Yinlingquan lies in the depression at the interior border of the medial epicondyle of the tibia, like a spring at the foot of a hill.

Location On the medial aspect of the lower leg, in the depression between the lower border of the medial condyle of the tibia and medial aspect of the tibia.

Indications Yinlingquan is a key point to fortify the spleen and drain the water, it can treat acute or chronic enteritis, bacterial dysentery, urinary retention, incontinence, urinary tract infection, vaginitis, lower extremity edema, disorders of knee and its surrounding soft tissues.

Methods Press and rub Yinlingquan point clockwise for 2 minutes with the pulp of thumb and then press it for 30 seconds until you feel sore. Moxibustion is also optional.

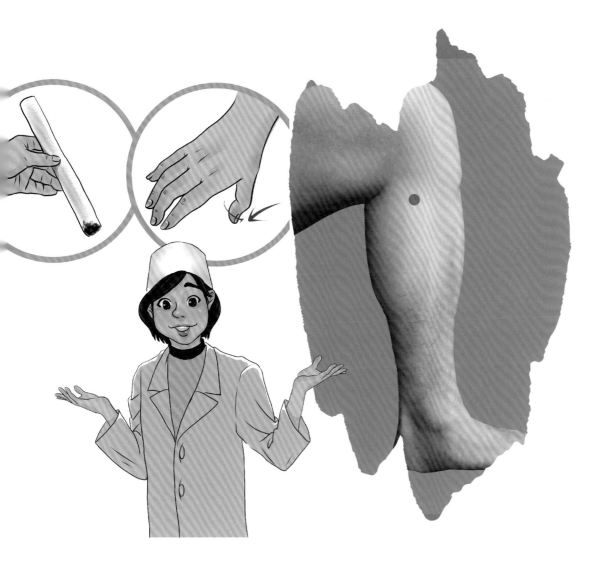

丰隆穴

来源　　　水湿云气传至本穴后，化雨而降，且降雨量大，如雷雨之轰隆有声，故名。

位置　　　位于人体的小腿前外侧，外踝尖上8寸，条口穴外1寸，距胫骨前缘2横指（中指）。

主要作用　　　治疗耳源性眩晕、高血压、高脂血症、神经衰弱、精神分裂症、支气管炎、腓肠肌痉挛、肥胖症等。本穴位是"化痰要穴"，尤其适宜于脾虚生痰的证型。

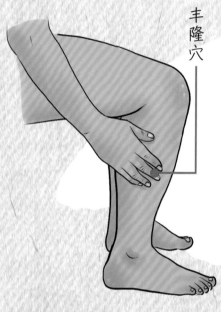

丰隆穴

始点

操作方法

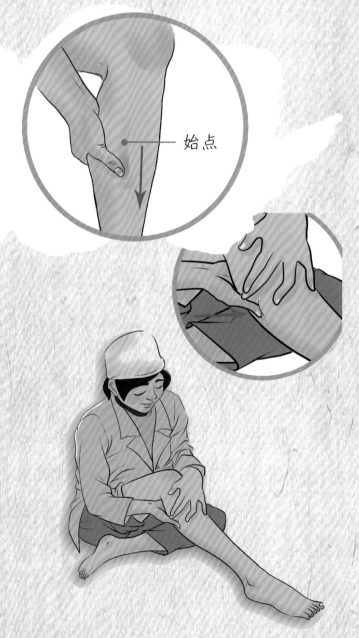

用大拇指点按丰隆穴3分钟，然后沿顺时针揉丰隆穴10分钟，后用大拇指沿丰隆穴向下单方向搓（即只能是由丰隆穴向下，而不能是由丰隆穴向下然后由下到上这样地来回搓）10分钟即可。也可用艾条温和灸的方法。

Fenglong Point (ST40)

Nomenclature The plentiful damp wind qi of the Stomach Meridian flows to this point and transforms into rain. Large rain falls with rumbling thunder.

Location On the anterior aspect of the lower leg, 8 cun superior to the external malleolus, lateral to ST38, two finger-breadth (middle finger) from the anterior crest of the tibia.

Indications Fenglong point can be used to treat otogenic vertigo, hypertension, hyperlipidemia, neurasthenia, schizophrenia, bronchitis, gastrocnemius spasm and obesity. As a key point for reducing phlegm, Fenglong is especially effective in treating phlegm caused by spleen deficiency.

Methods Press Fenglong points with thumbs for 3 minutes, rub it clockwise for 10 minutes and then downwards for 10 minutes. Moxibustion is also optional.

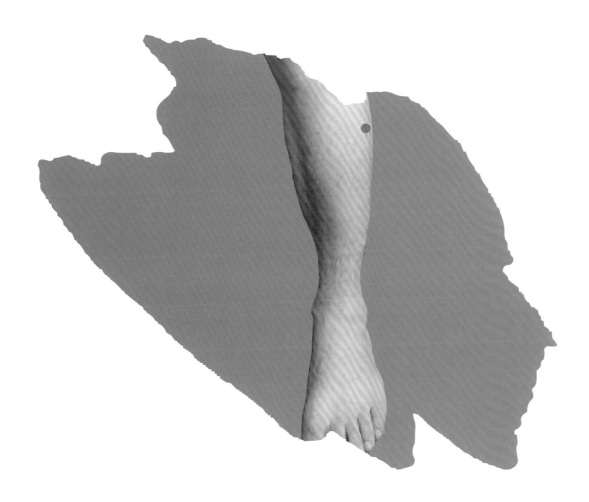

承山穴

来　源	意指随膀胱经经水下行沉降的脾土堆积如大山之状。
位　置	微微施力踮起脚尖，小腿后侧肌肉浮起的尾端即为承山穴。
主要作用	为治疗小腿抽筋、小腿酸痛等症状，及便秘、脱肛、痔疮等肛门疾患的常用效穴。

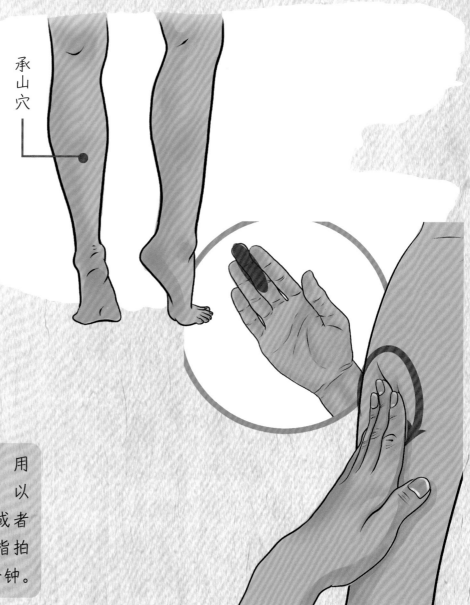

承山穴

操作方法

按揉或拍打。用同侧手四指并拢，以中指指腹按揉，或者用同侧并拢的手指拍打，每次2～3分钟。

Chengshan Point (BL57)

Nomenclature Soil of spleen goes downward along water of Bladder Meridian and deposits here like a mountain.

Location On the posterior midline of the leg, midway between Weizhong (BL40) and Kunlun (BL60), in the depression formed between the gastrocnemius muscle bellies when lifting the heel.

Indications Chengshan is an effective point for leg spasm and pain, and anal disorders such as constipation, rectocele, hemorrhoids.

Methods Press and rub Chengshan with the pulp of middle finger (four fingers close to each other) for 2 to 3 minutes. Or, pat the point with four fingers together for 2 to 3 minutes.

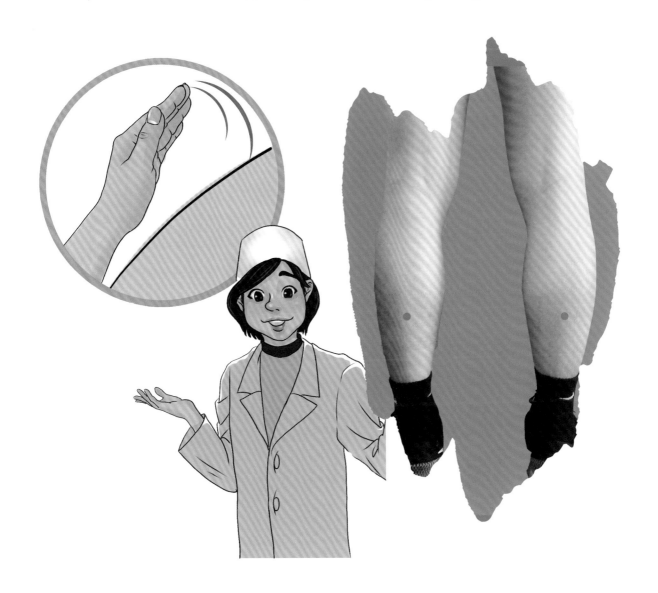

三阴交穴

来　源	意指足部的肝、脾、肾三条阴经中气血物质在本穴交会。
位　置	在内踝尖直上 3 寸，胫骨后缘。
主要作用	主治月经不调、不孕症、遗精、阳痿、遗尿、湿疹、失眠等。

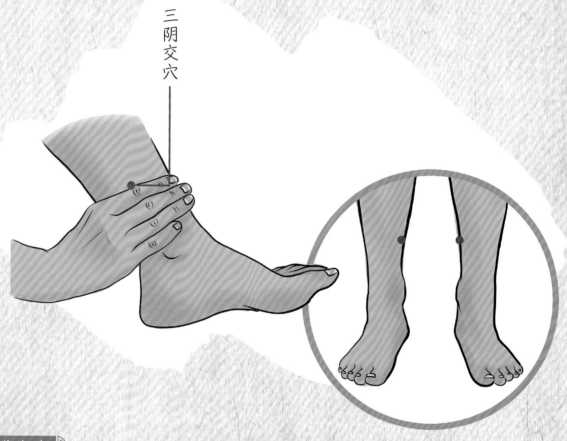

三阴交穴

操作方法

每天晚上 9 点 ~ 11 点，三焦经当令之时，用拇指或食指指端按揉两条腿的三阴交各 15 分钟。

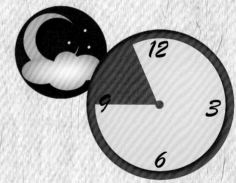

Sanyinjiao Point (SP6)

Nomenclature Sanyinjiao is an intersecting point of Spleen Meridian, Liver Meridian and Kidney Meridian.

Location On the medial aspect of the lower leg, 3 cun above the medial malleolus, on the posterior border of the medial aspect of the tibia.

Indications Irregular menstruation, infertility, spermatorrhea, impotence, enuresis, eczema, insomnia.

Methods Choose to have tuina at 9 to 11 o' clock in the evening. Press and rub Sanyinjiao points with thumbs or index fingers for 15 minutes.

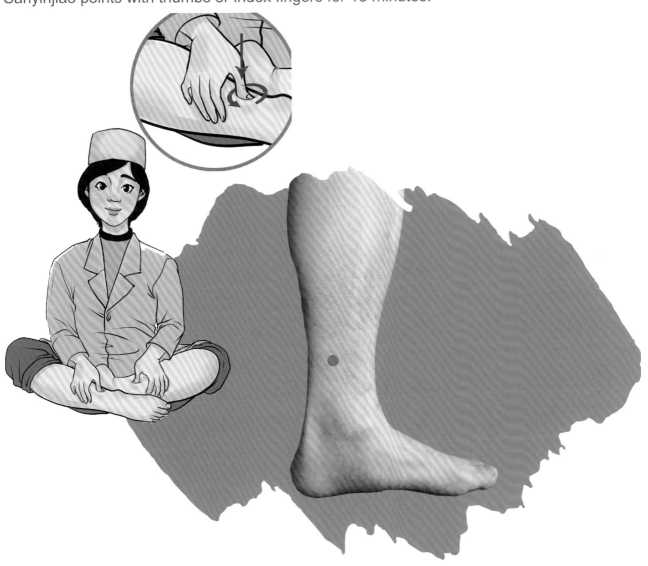

太溪穴

| 来　源 | 意指肾经水液在此形成较大的溪水。 |

| 位　置 | 正坐，平放足底，太溪穴位于足内侧，内踝后方与脚跟骨筋腱之间的凹陷处。 |

| 主要作用 | 为补肾要穴，可治疗头痛，眩晕，咽喉肿痛，齿痛，耳鸣，耳聋，气喘，糖尿病，失眠，健忘，腰脊酸痛，下肢凉，小便频数，以及男性女性生殖问题如月经不调、遗精、阳痿等。 |

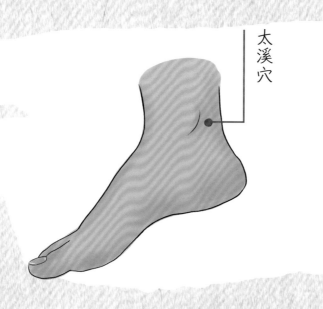

太溪穴

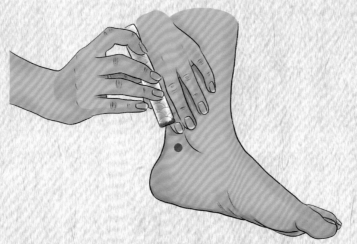

操作方法

按揉，用手拇指指腹按揉脚的太溪穴，每次2~3分钟。也可以用艾灸温和灸的方法，每穴灸5分钟左右。

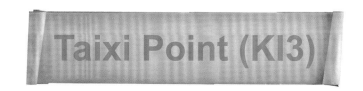

Taixi Point (KI3)

Nomenclature Water in Kidney Meridian flows here and becomes a larger stream.

Location On the medial aspect of the foot, posterior to the medial malleolus, in the depression between the tip of the medial malleolus and achilles tendon.

Indications Taixi is a key point for tonifying kidney. It can treat headache, dizziness, sore throat, toothache, tinnitus, deafness, asthma, diabetes, insomnia, forgetfulness, lumbar pain and soreness, cold lower limbs, frequent micturition, reproductive problems like irregular menstruation, spermatorrhea and impotence.

Methods Press and rub Taixi with the pulp of the thumb for 2 to 3 minutes. Besides, moxibustion for 5 minutes is also useful.

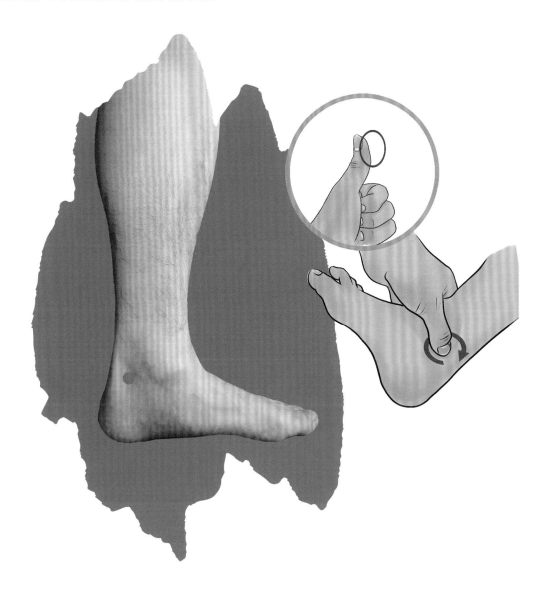

涌泉穴

来　源　肾经之气犹如源泉之水，来源于足下，涌出灌溉周身各处，故名涌泉。

位　置　在人体足底，位于足前部凹陷处，第2、第3趾趾缝纹头端与足跟连线的前三分之一处。

主要作用　防治老年性的哮喘、腰腿酸软无力、失眠多梦、神经衰弱、头晕、头痛、高血压、耳聋、耳鸣、大便秘结等。

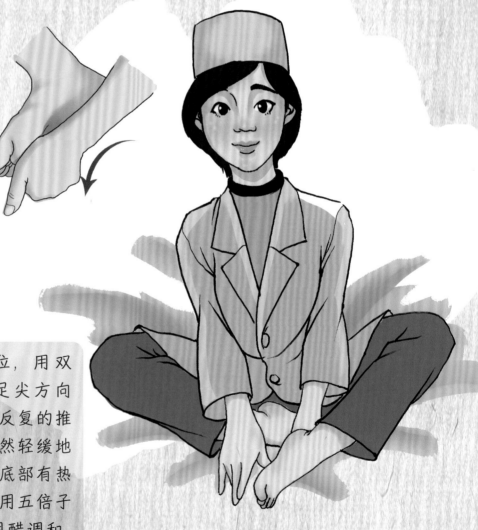

操作方法

在床上取坐位，用双手拇指从足跟向足尖方向推按涌泉穴处，做反复的推搓；或用双手掌自然轻缓地拍打涌泉穴，以足底部有热感为适宜。也可以用五倍子5～10克研末，用醋调和，巴布膏贴脚心，治疗失眠。

Yongquan Point (KI1)

Nomenclature   The qi of Kidney Meridian comes from the sole and flows upwards to whole body like a gushing spring.

Location   On the sole, in the depression when the foot is in plantar flexion, approximately at the anterior third and the posterior two thirds of the line from the web between the 2nd and 3rd toes to the back of the heel.

Indications   Yongquan point can treat senile asthma, weakness in waist and leg, insomnia, dreaminess, neurasthenia, dizziness, headache, hypertension, deafness, tinnitus, constipation and so on.

Methods   Rub or push Yongquan point in the direction from heel to toes repeatedly while sitting on the bed. Or, pat the point gently until the area becomes warm. To treat insomnia, stir gallnut powders (5 to 10 g) with vinegar and then cover them on the sole.

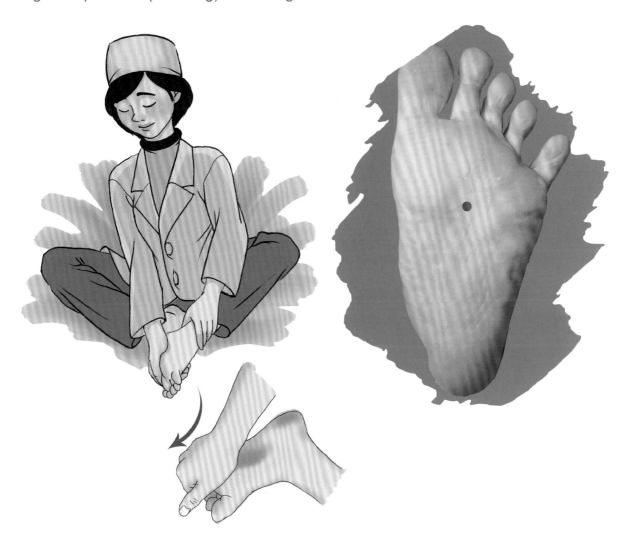

81